THE WAY TO LOCATE ACU-POINTS

Edited by
Associate Professor Yang Jiasan
Translated by
Dr. Meng Xiankun and Dr. Li Xuewu
Advised by
Associate Professor He Meisheng

FOREIGN LANGUAGES PRESS
BEIJING

First Edition 1982
Second Printing 1988
Third Printing 1998

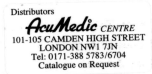

Distributors
AcuMedic CENTRE
101-105 CAMDEN HIGH STREET
LONDON NW1 7JN
Tel: 0171-388 5783/6704
Catalogue on Request

ISBN 7-119-00669-X
© Foreign Languages Press, Beijing, China, 1982
Published by Foreign Languages Press
24 Baiwanzhuang Road, Beijing 100037, China

Distributed by China International Book Trading Corporation
35 Chegongzhuang Xilu, Beijing 100044, China
P.O. Box 399, Beijing, China

Printed in the People's Republic of China

CONTENTS

PREFACE

Acupuncture and moxibustion has a history of several thousand years in treating diseases by the Chinese people.

To locate the points properly is the key step in acupuncture therapy, it is a significant in obtaining a satisfactory therapeutic effect. Therefore, it is of prime importance for those who learn acupuncture to have a thorough training in the basic skill of locating points.

Dr. Yang Jiasan, associate professor and head of the Acupuncture Department of Dongzhimen Hospital, has been engaged both in clinical and teaching work for several decades. He has a deep understanding of the classical and modern books on acupuncture. After a long study and repeated practice, he has developed a method of locating points, known as "Locating points by dividing the body and the channels into parts and according to anatomical landmarks."

Professor Yang's experience of locating points is taking anatomical landmarks for criterion as much as possible. Points of several channels adjacent to one another are grouped together according to different areas of the body. Such way to locate points is simple and easy to understand. Being concise and practical, it is very suitable both for teaching and clinical work.

Dr. Geng Enguang and Zhou Jiangchuan give assistance to author in writing the book. Thank them for their help.

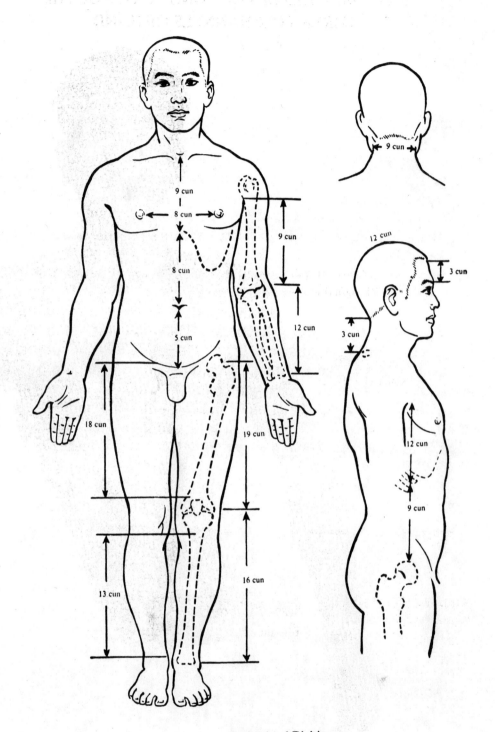

Proportional Division

I. THE METHOD OF LOCATING POINTS OF THE THREE YIN CHANNELS OF HAND

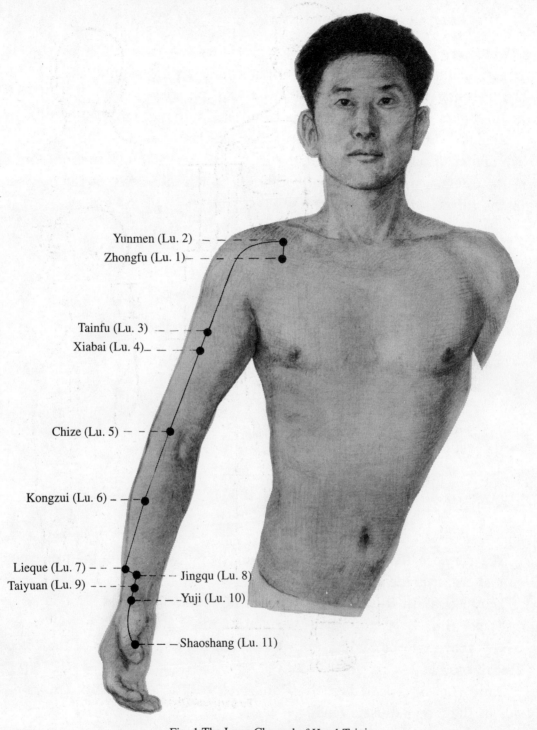

Yunmen (Lu. 2)

Zhongfu (Lu. 1)

Tainfu (Lu. 3)

Xiabai (Lu. 4)

Chize (Lu. 5)

Kongzui (Lu. 6)

Lieque (Lu. 7)

Taiyuan (Lu. 9)

Jingqu (Lu. 8)

Yuji (Lu. 10)

Shaoshang (Lu. 11)

Fig. 1 The Lung Channel of Hand-Taiyin

They start from the chest and run to the hand.

1. The Lung Channel of Hand-Taiyin

The Lung Channel of Hand-Taiyin originates at point Zhongfu (Lu. 1). It goes along the anterior border of the radius on the medial aspect of the arm, passing through the cubital fossa and the wrist joint. Then it ends at the radial side of the tip of the thumb (Shaoshang, Lu. 11).

Zhongfu (Lu. 1): 1 *cun* directly below Yunmen (Lu. 2).

Yunmen (Lu. 2): Level with the lower border of the sternal extremity of the clavicle, two finger-breadths lateral to the mid-point of the clavicle, in the infraclavicular fossa. (See Fig. 2)

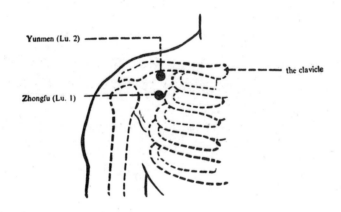

Fig. 2 Yunmen and Zhongfu

The distance from the anterior end of the axillary fold to the transverse cubital crease is measured as 9 *cun*.

Tianfu (Lu. 3): 3 *cun* below the end of the axillary fold.

Xiabai (Lu. 4): 4 *cun* below the end of the axillary fold.

The above two points are both located in the radial sulcus of the biceps brachii muscle.

Chize (Lu. 5): Located in the transverse cubital crease, on the radial side of the biceps muscle tendon.

The distance between the distal skin crease of the wrist to the transverse cubital crease is measured as 12 *cun*.

Kongzui (Lu. 6): 7 *cun* above the distal wrist crease, on the medial border of the radius.

Lieque (Lu. 7): At the origin of the styloid process of the radius, 1.5 *cun* proximal to the wrist crease.

Jingqu (Lu. 8): On the medial side of the styloid process of the radius, level with the highest spot.

Taiyuan (Lu. 9): On the distal crease of the wrist, at the lower border of the trapezium on the radial side.

Yuji (Lu. 10): Proximal to the metacarpophalangeal joint of the thumb, on the radial border of the metacarpal bone.

Shaoshang (Lu. 11): On the radial side of the thumb, about 0.1 *cun* from the corner of the nail.

How to locate the points of this channel?

On the borders of the bone;

Adjacent to the tendon;

In the sulcus.

On the borders of the bone: Kongzui (Lu. 6) on the medial border of the radius, Jingqu (Lu. 8) on the medial border of the styloid process of the radius.

Adjacent to the tendon: Chize (Lu. 5) in the elbow crease, at the radial side of the tendon of biceps brachii.

In the sulcus: Tianfu (Lu. 3) and Xiabai (Lu. 4) in the radial sulcus of the biceps brachii muscle.

2. The Heart Channel of Hand-Shaoyin

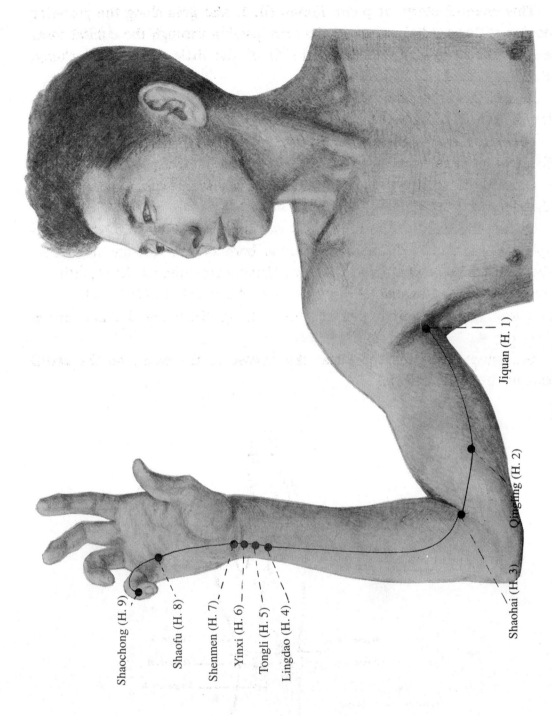

Shaochong (H. 9)

Shaofu (H. 8)

Shenmen (H. 7)

Yinxi (H. 6)

Tongli (H. 5)

Lingdao (H. 4)

Shaohai (H. 3)

Qingling (H. 2)

Jiquan (H. 1)

Fig. 3 The Heart Channel of Hand-Shaoyin

The Heart Channel of Hand-Shaoyin:

This channel starts at point Jiquan (H. 1) and goes along the posterior border of the medial aspect of the arm, passing through the cubital fossa and the wrist, it ends at the medial side of the little finger (Shaochong, H. 9).

Jiquan (H. 1): In the centre of the armpit, on the medial side of axillary artery.

Qingling (H. 2): 3 *cun* above the medial epicondyle of the humerus, in the groove of the biceps brachii muscle on the ulnar aspect.

Shaohai (H. 3): At the medial end of the transverse cubital crease when the elbow is flexed.

Taking the head of the ulnar as 1 *cun* and draw three parallel lines respectively along its distal and proximal borders and through its centre. On the radial side of the tendon of m. flexor carpi ulnaris, level with the proximal line is Lingdao (H. 4); level with the middle line is Tongli (H. 5); and level with the distal line is Yinxi (H. 6). They are 0.5 *cun* apart. (See Fig. 4)

Shenmen (H. 7): At the distal skin crease of the wrist, on the radial side of the pisiform bone.

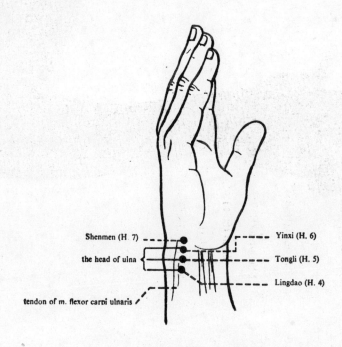

Fig. 4 Head of Ulna as Landmark

Shaofu (H. 8): Between the 4th and 5th metacarpal bone, posterior to the metacarpophalangeal joints, on the transverse crease of the palm.

Shaochong (H. 9): On the radial side of the tip of the little finger, about 0.1 *cun* posterior to the corner of the nail.

How to locate the points of this channel?

Find them in the groove;

Adjacent to the tendon;

At the end of the crease.

In the groove: Qingling (H. 2) in the groove of the biceps brachii muscle on the ulnar aspect.

Adjacent to the tendon: Lingdao (H. 4), Tongli (H. 5), Yinxi (H. 6) and Shenmen (H. 7) on the radial side of the tendon of m. flexor carpi ulnaris.

At the end of the crease: Shaohai (H. 3) at the medial end of the transverse cubital crease when the elbow is flexed.

3. The Pericardium Channel of Hand-Jueyin

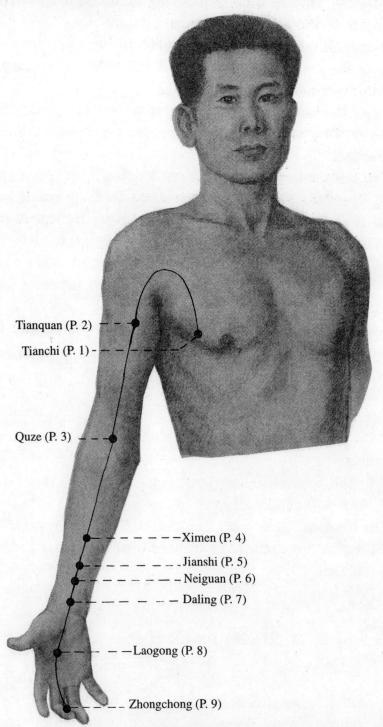

Tianquan (P. 2)

Tianchi (P. 1)

Quze (P. 3)

Ximen (P. 4)

Jianshi (P. 5)

Neiguan (P. 6)

Daling (P. 7)

Laogong (P. 8)

Zhongchong (P. 9)

Fig. 5 The Pericardium Channel of Hand-Jueyin

The Pericardium Channel of Hand-Jueyin: It starts at point Tianchi (P. 1) and goes along the medial aspect of the arm between the Lung and the Heart Channel, passing through the cubital fossa and the wrist, it ends at the tip of the middle finger (Zhongchong, P. 9).

Tianchi (P. 1): 1 *cun* lateral to the nipple, in the 4th intercostal space.

Tianquan (P. 2): 2 *cun* below the end of the anterior axillary fold, on the belly of m. biceps brachii.

Quze (P. 3): On the transverse cubital crease, on the ulnar side of the tendon of m. biceps brachii.

(The distance from the transverse cubital crease to the most distal skin crease of the wrist is measured as 12 *cun*.)

There are four points between the tendons of m. palmaris longus and m. flexor carpi radialis: Ximen (P. 4), 5 *cun* above the transverse crease of the wrist. Jianshi (P. 5), 3 *cun* above the wrist crease. Neiguan (P. 6), 2 *cun* above the wrist crease and Daling (P. 7) is right on the wrist crease.

Laogong (P. 8): On the radial side of the 3rd metacarpal bone, proximal to the metacarpophalangeal joint.

Zhongchong (P. 9): On the middle of the tip of the middle finger.

How to locate the points of this channel?

On the belly of the muscle;

Adjacent to the tendon;

At the cleft of the tendons.

On the belly of the muscle: Tianquan (P. 2) is located on the belly of m. biceps brachii.

Adjacent to the tendon: Quze (P. 3) is located at the ulnar side of the tendon of m. biceps brachii.

Cleft of the tendons: Ximen (P. 4), Jianshi (P. 5), Neiguan (P. 6), and Daling (P. 7) are on the cleft of the tendons of m. palmaris longus and m. flexor carpi radialis.

4. **The Summing-up of Locating Points of the Three Yin Channels of Hand**

Points according to the different parts of the body.

1. The finger tip region: Points are located at the tip of the finger or the roots and corners of the nails.

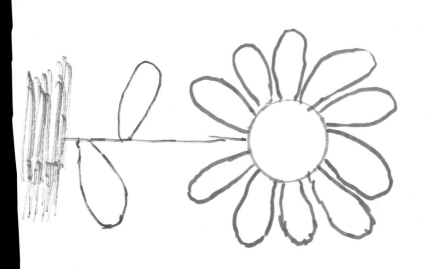

Shaochong (H. 9): About 0.1 *cun* proximal to the corner of the nail, on the radial side of the little finger.

Zhongchong (P. 9): Midpoint of the tip of the middle finger.

Shaoshang (Lu. 11): About 0.1 *cun* proximal to the corner of the nail, on the radial side of the thumb.

Shaochong (H. 9) and Shaoshang (Lu. 11) are all located at the root of the nail. They are not level with the nail. (See Fig. 6)

2. The palm region: The points are located posteriorly to the metacarpophalangeal joints.

Yuji (Lu. 11): Posterior to the metacarpophalangeal joint of the thumb, on the medial side of the first metacarpal bone.

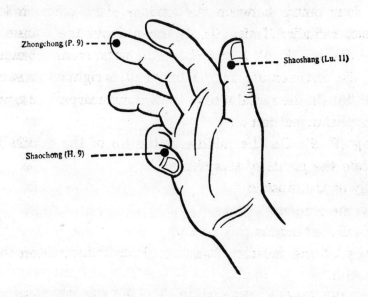

Fig. 6 Points at Finger Tips and Nail Corners

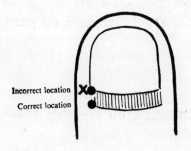

Fig. 7 How to Locate Point at Nail Corner

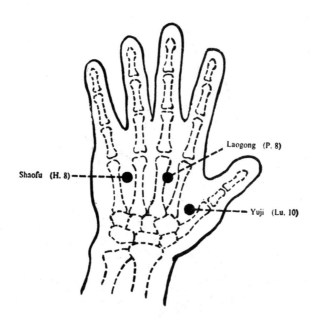

Fig. 8 Points Posterior to Metacarpophalangeal Joint

Laogong (P. 8): Posterior to the 3rd metacarpophalangeal joint, on the radial side of the 3rd metacarpal bone, on the transverse palmar crease.

Shaofu (H. 8): Between the 4th and 5th metacarpal bones, posteriorly to the metacarpophalangeal joints, on the transverse palmar crease.

3. The wrist region: The points are located on the transverse crease and between two bones and two tendons.

The transverse crease refers to the distal skin crease of the wrist.

The two bones refer to the pisiform bone and the trapezium.

The two tendons are the tendons of the palmaris longus muscle and flexor carpi radialis muscle.

Taiyuan (Lu. 9): Inferior border of the trapezium, at the radial side.

Shenmen (H. 7): Radial side of the pisiform bone.

Daling (P. 7): Between the two tendons.

These three points are all on the distal skin crease of the wrist. (See Fig. 9)

4. The forearm region: The points are on the border of the bone, beside the tendon, or between the tendons.

The bone is the radius.

Jingqu (Lu. 8): On the radial border of the styloid process of the radius, level with the highest spot.

Kongzui (Lu. 6): On the ulnar border of the radius, 7 *cun* above the distal skin crease of the wrist. (See Fig. 10)

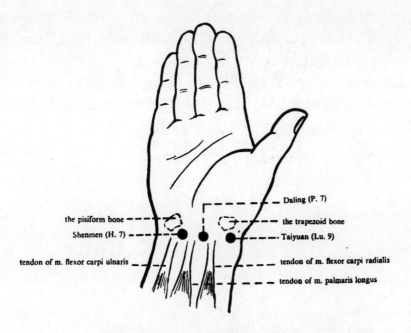

the pisiform bone ------ Daling (P. 7)

the pisiform bone -----
Shenmen (H. 7) -----

----- the trapezoid bone
----- Taiyuan (Lu. 9)

tendon of m. flexor carpi ulnaris -----

----- tendon of m. flexor carpi radialis
----- tendon of m. palmaris longus

Fig. 9 Two Bones, Two Tendons and a Transverse Crease as Landmarks

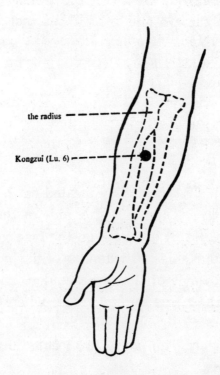

the radius -----

Kongzui (Lu. 6) -----

Fig. 10   Point at Edge of Radius

Adjacent to the tendon e.g. Shenmen (H. 7), Yinxi (H. 6), Tongli (H. 5) and Lingdao (H. 4) are located on the radial side of the tendon of the flexor carpi ulnaris muscle.

Between the tendons e.g. Daling (P. 7), Neiguan (P. 6), Jianshi (P. 5) and Ximen (P. 4) are located between the tendons of m. palmaris longus and m. flexor carpi radialis. (See Fig. 11)

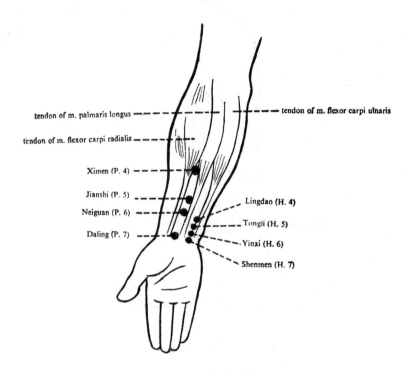

Fig. 11 Points Between and Along Tendons

5.   The cubital region: The points are located on the transverse cubital crease, at the end of the crease and on either side of the tendon.

Chize (Lu. 5) and Quze (P. 3) are both on the transverse cubital crease. Chize (Lu. 5) is on the radial side of the tendon of the biceps brachii muscle. Quze (P. 3) is on the ulnar side of the same tendon. Shaohai (H. 3) is at the medial end of the transverse cubital crease when the elbow is flexed. (See Fig. 12 and Fig. 13)

6.   The upper arm region: The points are located on the biceps brachii muscle and its two grooves.

Tianquan (P. 2) is in between the two heads of the biceps brachii muscle, 2 *cun* below the end of the axillary fold. Tianfu (Lu. 3) is in the groove of the biceps brachii muscle on the radial side, 3 *cun* below the end of the axillary fold. Xiabai (Lu. 4) is in the same groove, 4 *cun* below the end of the axillary fold. Qingling (H. 2) is in the groove of the same muscle on the ulnar side, 3 *cun* above the medial epicondyle of the humerus. (See Fig. 14)

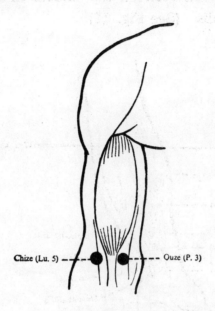

Chize (Lu. 5) — — — — —   — — — Ouze (P. 3)

Fig. 12 Points at Both Sides of Tendon

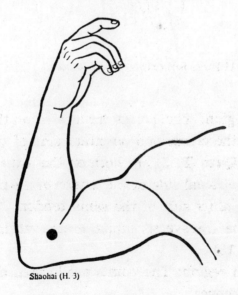

Shaohai (H. 3)

Fig. 13 Point at End of Elbow Crease

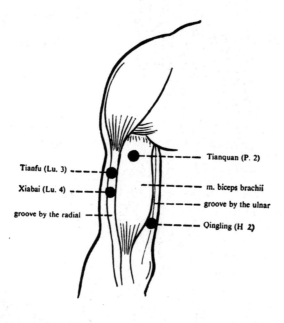

Tianfu (Lu. 3)

Xiabai (Lu. 4)

groove by the radial

Tianquan (P. 2)

m. biceps brachii

groove by the ulnar

Qingling (H 2)

Fig. 14 A Muscle and Two Grooves as Landmarks

II. THE METHOD OF LOCATING POINTS OF THE THREE YANG CHANNELS OF HAND

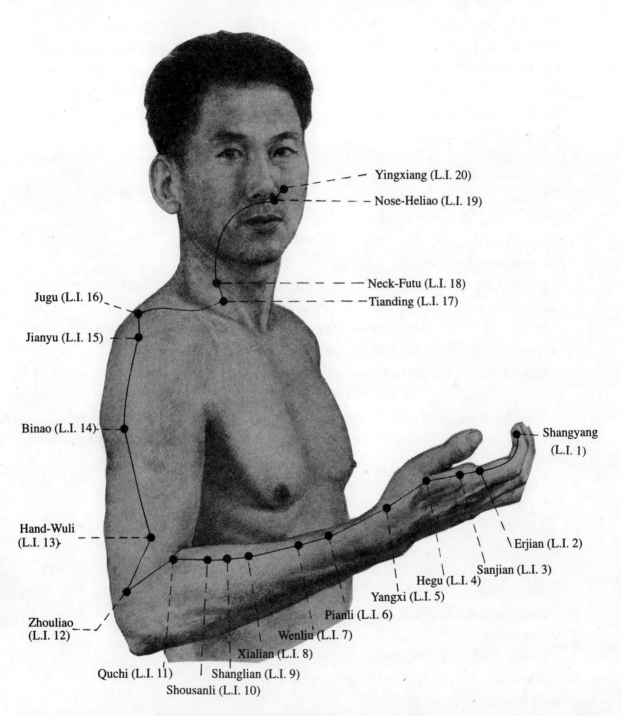

Fig. 15 The Large Intestine Channel of Hand-Yangming

The three Yang Channels of Hand run from the hand to the head.

1. The Large Intestine Channel of Hand-Yangming

The Large Intestine Channel of Hand-Yangming originates from Shang-yang (L. I. 1) and runs upward along the anterior border of the lateral aspect of the upper limb, passing through the wrist and elbow and up to the shoulder joint. There, it further ascends to the neck and the facial region, terminating at the lateral side of the nose, Yingxiang (L. I. 20). (See Fig. 15)

Shangyang (L. I. 1): On the radial side of the index finger, about 0.1 *cun* posterior to the corner of the nail.

Erjian (L. I. 2): On the radial side of the index finger, distal to the metacarpophalangeal joint.

Sanjian (L. I. 3): On the radial side of the index finger, proximal to the metacarpophalangeal joint.

Hegu (L. I. 4): Midway between the junction of the 1st and 2nd meta-carpal bones and the margin of the web.

Yangxi (L. I. 5): On the wrist between the two tendons (the tendons of m. extensor pollicis brevis and extensor pollicis longus).

Quchi (L. I. 11): At the external end of the cubital crease when the elbow is flexed, on the medial aspect of the radius.

The distance between Yangxi (L. I. 5) and Quchi (L. I. 11) is 12 *cun*.

Pianli (L. I. 6): 3 *cun* above Yangxi (L. I. 5), on the lateral aspect of the radius.

Wenliu (L. I. 7): 5 *cun* above Yangxi (L. I. 5), on the lateral aspect of the radius.

Xialian (L. I. 8): 4 *cun* below Quchi (L. I. 11), on the lateral aspect of the radius.

Shanglian (L. I. 9): 3 *cun* below Quchi (L. I. 11), on the medial aspect of the radius.

Shousanli (L. I. 10): 2 *cun* below Quchi (L. I. 11), on the medial aspect of the radius.

Quchi (L. I. 11): See above.

Zhouliao (L. I. 12): 1 *cun* above the lateral epicondyle of the humerus, on the lateral border of it.

Hand-Wuli (L. I. 13): 3 *cun* above the lateral epicondyle, on the medial border of the humerus.

Binao (L. I. 14): On the lower border of the deltoid muscle and the medial side of the humerus.

Jianyu (L. I. 15): Directly below the anterior border of the acromion, where a depression is formed when the arm is abducted.

Jugu (L. I. 16): At the depression between the acromial extremity of the clavicle and the spine of the scapula.

Tianding (L. I. 17): 1 *cun* above the middle of the supraclavicular fossa, at the posterior margin of the sternocleidomastoid muscle.

Neck-Futu (L. I. 18): At the level of Adam's apple, just between the two heads of the sternocleidomastoid muscle.

Nose-Heliao (L. I. 19): Directly below the lateral margin of the nostril, level with Renzhong (Du. 26).

Yingxiang (L. I. 20): In the nasolabial sulcus, at the level of the midpoint of the lateral border of ala nasi.

How to locate the points of this channel?

Find them at the sides of the bone.

Quchi (L. I. 11), Shousanli (L. I. 10) and Shanglian (L. I. 9) are on the medial aspect of the radius, while Xialian (L. I. 8), Wenliu (L. I. 7) and Pianli (L. I. 6) are on its lateral aspect. Zhouliao (L. I. 12) is on the lateral aspect of the humerus. Hand-Wuli (L. I. 13) and Binao (L. I. 14) are on its medial aspect. These points are located with the elbow flexed.

2. The Small Intestine Channel of Hand-Taiyang

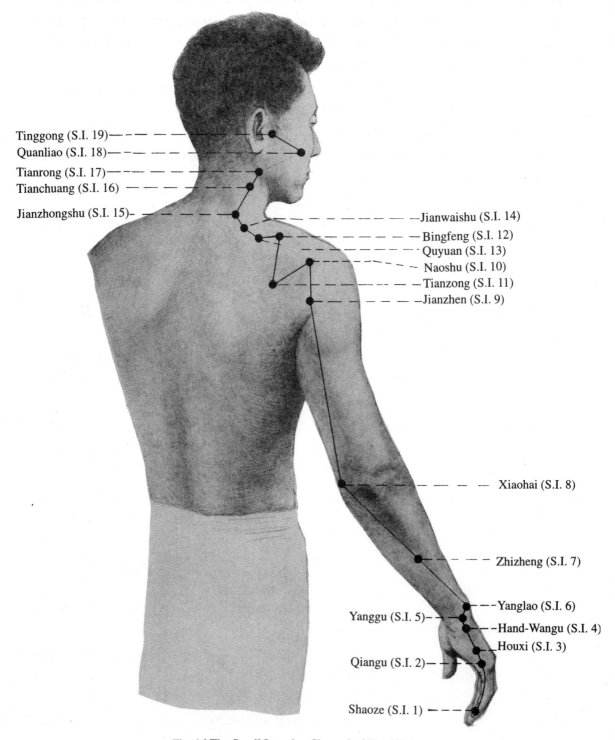

Tinggong (S.I. 19)

Quanliao (S.I. 18)

Tianrong (S.I. 17)

Tianchuang (S.I. 16)

Jianzhongshu (S.I. 15)

Jianwaishu (S.I. 14)

Bingfeng (S.I. 12)

Quyuan (S.I. 13)

Naoshu (S.I. 10)

Tianzong (S.I. 11)

Jianzhen (S.I. 9)

Xiaohai (S.I. 8)

Zhizheng (S.I. 7)

Yanglao (S.I. 6)

Yanggu (S.I. 5)

Hand-Wangu (S.I. 4)

Houxi (S.I. 3)

Qiangu (S.I. 2)

Shaoze (S.I. 1)

Fig. 16 The Small Intestine Channel of Hand-Taiyang

The Small Intestine Channel of Hand-Taiyang starts from the ulnar side of the tip of the little finger at Shaoze (S. I. 1) and runs upward along the posterior border of the lateral aspect of the upper limb, passing through the wrist and elbow and up to the scapula, then it ascends to the neck and cheek, terminating at Tinggong (S. I. 19).

Shaoze (S. I. 1): On the ulnar side of the little finger, about 0.1 *cun* proximal to the corner of the nail.

Qiangu (S. I. 2) and Houxi (S. I. 3):

Distal to the metacarpophalangeal joint is Qiangu (S. I. 2), and that proximal to it is Houxi (S. I. 3).

Hand-Wangu (S. I. 4) and Yanggu (S. I. 5):

Distal to the hamate bone is Hand-Wangu (S. I. 4), and that proximal to it is Yanggu (S. I. 5).

Shaoze (S. I. 1), Qiangu (S. I. 2), Houxi (S. I. 3), Hand-Wangu (S. I. 4) and Yanggu (S. I. 5) are all on the junction of the red and white skin.

Yanglao (S. I. 6): On the head of the ulnar where there is a seam when the palm turns to the chest.

Zhizheng (S. I. 7): 5 *cun* above the wrist, on the border of the ulna.

Xiaohai (S. I. 8): In the fossa between the ulnar olecranon and the medial epicondyle of the humerus.

Jianzhen (S. I. 9): 1 *cun* above the posterior end of the axillary fold.

Naoshu (S. I. 10): Straightly above Jianzhen (S. I. 9), in the depression below the spine of the scapula.

Taking the spine of the scapula as landmark for locating the points:

Tianzong (S. I. 11): 1 *cun* below the midpoint of the lower border of the spine.

Bingfeng (S. I. 12): 1 *cun* above the midpoint of the upper border of the spine.

Quyuan (S. I. 13): On the upper border of the spine, 1 *cun* lateral to its medial end.

Jianwaishu (S. I. 14): 3 *cun* from Taodao (Du. 13), which is below the spinous process of the 1st thoracic vertebra.

Jianzhongshu (S. I. 15): 2 *cun* from Dazhui (Du. 14), which is below the spinous process of the 7th cervical vertebra.

Tianchuang (S. I. 16): Level with the laryngeal prominence, on the posterior border of the sternocleidomastoid muscle.

Tianrong (S. I. 17): Level with the angle of the mandible, on the anterior border of the sternocleidomastoid muscle.

Quanliao (S. I. 18): On the lower border of the zygomatic bone, directly below the external canthus.

Tinggong (S. I. 19): Anterior to the tragus, where a depression is formed when the mouth is opened.

How to locate the points of this channel?

Look for them on the superior or inferior border of the scapular spine. Bingfeng (S. I. 12) 1 *cun* above the midpoint of the upper border of the scapular spine. Tianzong (S. I. 11) 1 *cun* below the midpoint of the lower border of the scapular spine. Naoshu (S. I. 10) on the lower border of the scapular spine, 1 *cun* medial to its lateral end. Quyuan (S. I. 13) on the upper border of the scapular spine, 1 *cun* lateral to its medial end.

3. The Sanjiao Channel of Hand-Shaoyang

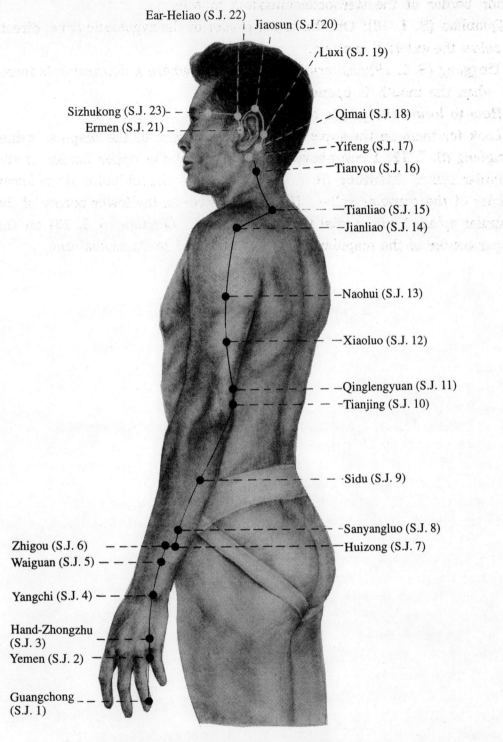

Ear-Heliao (S.J. 22)
Jiaosun (S.J. 20)
Luxi (S.J. 19)
Sizhukong (S.J. 23)
Ermen (S.J. 21)
Qimai (S.J. 18)
Yifeng (S.J. 17)
Tianyou (S.J. 16)
Tianliao (S.J. 15)
Jianliao (S.J. 14)
Naohui (S.J. 13)
Xiaoluo (S.J. 12)
Qinglengyuan (S.J. 11)
Tianjing (S.J. 10)
Sidu (S.J. 9)
Sanyangluo (S.J. 8)
Zhigou (S.J. 6)
Huizong (S.J. 7)
Waiguan (S.J. 5)
Yangchi (S.J. 4)
Hand-Zhongzhu (S.J. 3)
Yemen (S.J. 2)
Guangchong (S.J. 1)

Fig. 17 The Sanjiao Channel of Hand-Shaoyang

The. Sanjiao Channel of Hand-Shaoyang starts from the ulnar side of the tip of the ring finger at Guanchong (S. J. 1) and runs upward along the lateral aspect of the arm between the Small Intestine Channel and the Large Intestine Channel. It reaches the shoulder, ascends to the neck, winds around the ear and ends at Sizhukong (S. J. 23).

Guanchong (S. J. 1): On the ulnar side of the ring finger, about 0.1 *cun* posterior to the corner of the nail.

Yemen (S. J. 2) and Hand-Zhongzhu (S. J. 3): Yemen (S. J. 2) is distal to the metacarpophalangeal joint proximal to the metacarpophalangeal joint is Hand-Zhongzhu (S. J. 3).

Yangchi (S. J. 4): On the dorsum of the wrist, directly above the ring finger and between two tendons (The tendon of m. digitiquinti proprius and the tendon of m. extensor digitorum (communis).

Waiguan (S. J. 5): 2 *cun* above Yangchi (S. J. 4), between the ulnar and radius.

Zhigou (S. J. 6): 3 *cun* above Yangchi (S. J. 4), between the ulnar and radius.

Huizong (S. J. 7): 3 *cun* above Yangchi (S. J. 4), on the radial side of the ulnar.

Sanyangluo (S. J. 8): 4 *cun* above Yangchi (S. J. 4), between the ulnar and radius.

Sidu (S. J. 9): 7 *cun* above Yangchi (S. J. 4), between the ulnar and a radius.

Tianjing (S. J. 10): 1 *cun* above the olecranon, where a depression when the elbow is slightly flexed.

Qinglengyuan (S. J. 11): 2 *cun* above the olecranon.

Xiaoluo (S. J. 12) and Naohui (S. J. 13):

Naohui (S. J. 13) where the lower border of the deltoid muscle and the posterior border of the humerus meet. Midway between Qinglengyuan (S. J. 11) and Naohui (S. J. 13) is Xiaoluo (S. J. 12).

Jianliao (S. J. 14): In the depression where is directly below the posterior border of the acromial extremity of clavicle.

Tianliao (S. J. 15): The mediosuperior angle of the scapula.

Tianyou (S. J. 16): The posterior border of the sternocleidomastoid muscle, level with the angle of the mandible.

Yifeng (S. J. 17): On the midway between the mastoid process and the angle of the mandible.

Qimai (S. J. 18): On the antero-inferior aspect of the mastoid process.

Luxi (S. J. 19): On the antero-superior aspect of the mastoid process.

Jiaosun (S. J. 20): Fold the auricle it is level with the ear apex.

Ermen (S. J. 21): In the depression anterior to the supratragic notch.

Ear-Heliao (S. J. 22): 1 *cun* anterior to the root of the auricle.

Sizhukong (S. J. 23): In the depression at the lateral end of the eyebrow.

How to locate the points of this channel?

Between the ulna and the radius are Waiguan (S. J. 5), Zhigou (S. J. 6), Sanyangluo (S. J. 8) and Sidu (S. J. 9). Huizong (S. J. 7) is on the radial side of the ulnar, level with Zhigou (S. J. 6).

4.   The Summing-up of Locating Points in Three Yang Channels of Hand

1.   Finger tips: Points are located at the corners of nails.

Shangyang (L. I. 1): On the radial side of the index finger, proximal to the corner of the nail.

Guanchong (S. J. 1): On the ulnar side of the ring finger, proximal to the corner of the nail.

Shaoze (S. I. 1): On the ulnar side of the little finger, proximal to the corner of the nail. (See Fig. 18)

2.   Metacarpus: The points are located distally or proximally to metacarpophalangeal joints.

Erjian (L. I. 2) and Sanjian (L. I. 3) of the Large Intestine Channel: Distal and proximal to the 2nd metacarpophalangeal joint, on the radial side.

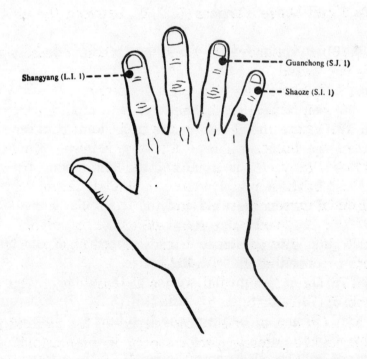

Fig. 18 Points Posterior to Nail Corners

Yemen (S. J. 2) and Hand-Zhongzhu (S. J. 3) of the Sanjiao Channel: Distal and proximal to the interspace between the 4th and 5th metacarpophalangeal joints.

Qiangu (S. I. 2) and Houxi (S. I. 3) of the Small Intestine Channel: Distal and proximal to the 5th metacarpophalangeal joint on the ulnar side. (See Fig. 19)

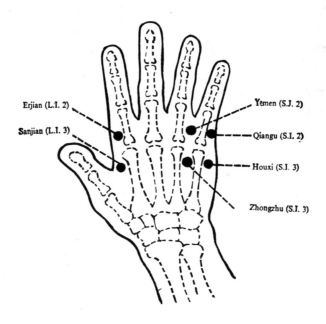

Fig. 19 Points Distal or Proximal to Metacarpophalangeal Joints

3.   Carpus: The points are located between the tendons or bones.

Yangxi (L. I. 5): On the radial side of the trapezium, between two tendons.

Yangchi (S. J. 4): Between the ulnar and the lunate bone, between two tendons.

Yanggu (S. I. 5): Between the ulna and the triangular bone. (See Fig. 20)

4.   Forearm: The points are located on the borders of the bones, between two bones or on either side of the bones.

Zhizheng (S. I. 6) is on the medial border of the ulna.

Waiguan (S. J. 5), Zhigou (S. J. 6), Huizong (S. J. 7), Sanyangluo (S. J. 8) and Sidu (S. J. 9) are all between the two bones. Huizong (S. J. 7) is on the radial side of the ulna.

Pianli (L. I. 6), Wenliu (L. I. 7) and Xialian (L. I. 8) are on the lateral side of the radius. Shanglian (L. I. 9), Shousanli (L. I. 10) and Quchi (L. I. 11) are on the medial side of the radius. (See Fig. 21)

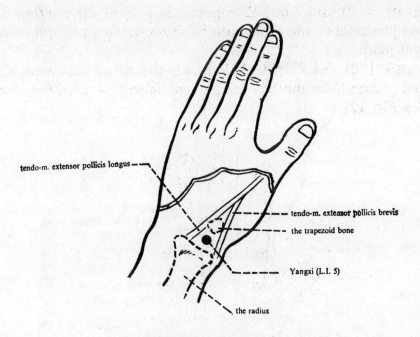

tendo-m. extensor pollicis longus

tendo-m. extensor pollicis brevis

the trapezoid bone

Yangxi (L.I. 5)

the radius

Fig. 20(1) Points Between Tendons or Bones

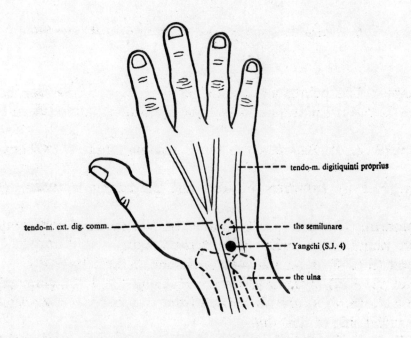

tendo-m. digitiquinti proprius

tendo-m. ext. dig. comm.

the semilunare

Yangchi (S.J. 4)

the ulna

Fig. 20(2) Points Between Tendons or Bones

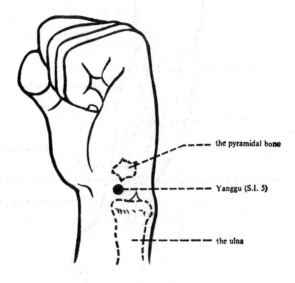

the pyramidal bone

Yanggu (S.I. 5)

the ulna

Fig. 20(3) Points Between Tendons or Bones

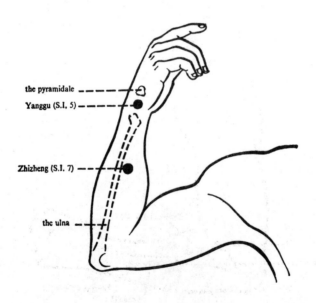

the pyramidale

Yanggu (S.I. 5)

Zhizheng (S.I. 7)

the ulna

Fig. 21(1) Points near the Bone

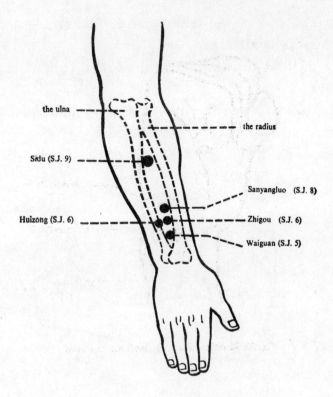

Fig. 21(2) Points Between Two Bones

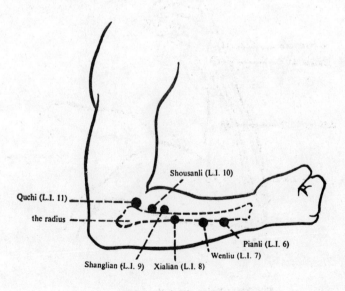

Fig. 21(3) Points on Both Sides of the Bone

5. Elbow: The end of the transverse cubital crease and the tip of the elbow are taken as landmarks.

Quchi (L. I. 11): At the external end of the cubital crease when the elbow is flexed.

Xiaohai (S. I. 8): Between the tip of the elbow and the medial epicondyle of the humerus.

Tianjing (S. J. 6): 1 *cun* above the tip of the elbow. (See Fig. 22)

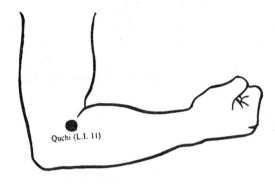

Fig. 22(1) Point at End of Elbow Crease

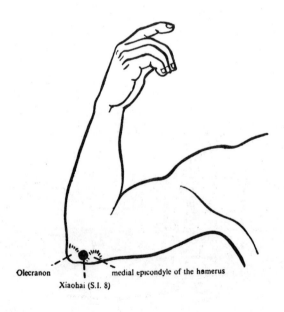

Fig. 22(2) Tip of Elbow as Landmark

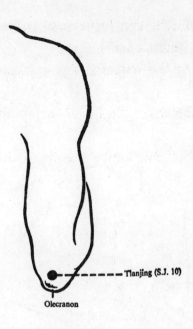

Fig. 22(3) Tip of Elbow as Landmark

6. Upper arm: The deltoid muscle and the humerus are taken as landmarks.

Binao (L. I. 14): Where the antero-inferior border of the deltoid muscle and the medial border of the humerus meet.

Naohui (S. J. 13): Where the postero-inferior border of the deltoid muscle and the lateral border of the humerus meet. (See Fig. 23)

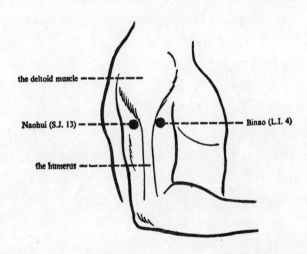

Fig. 23 Deltoid Muscle and Humerus as Landmarks

7. Shoulder joint: The points are located anteriorly or posteriorly to the acromial extremity of the clavicle.

In the depression directly below the acromial extremity of the clavicle and its anterior border is Jianyu (L. I. 15). Jianliao (S. J. 14) is in the depression directly below its posterior border. (See Fig. 24)

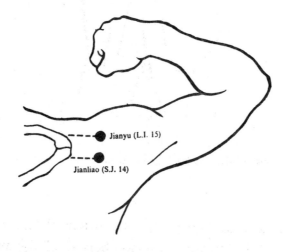

Fig. 24 Acromial Extremity of Clavicle as Landmark

8. Scapular region: The points are located superiorly or inferiorly to the midpoint or the two ends of the scapular spine.

Bingfeng (S. I. 12): 1 *cun* above the midpoint of the upper border of the scapular spine.

Tianzong (S. I. 11): 1 *cun* below the midpoint of the lower border of the scapular spine.

Naoshu (S. I. 10): On the lower border of the scapular spine, 1 *cun* medial to its lateral end.

Quyuan (S. I. 13): On the upper border of the scapular spine, 1 *cun* lateral to its medial end. (See Fig. 25)

9. Neck: The Adam's apple, the mandibular angle and the sterno-cleidomastoid muscle are taken as landmarks.

The points level with the Adam's apple:

Renying (St. 9): On the anterior border of the sternocleidomastoid muscle.

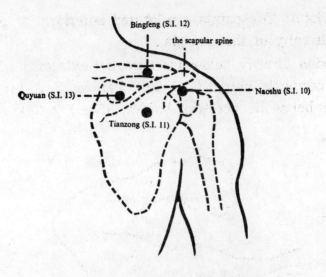

Fig. 25 Scapular Spine as Landmark

Neck-Futu (L. I. 18): Between the two heads of the muscle.
Tianchuang (S. I. 16): On the posterior border of the muscle.
Points level with the mandibular angle:
Tianrong (S. I. 17): On the anterior border of the muscle.
Tianyou (S. J. 16): On the posterior border of the muscle. (See Fig. 26)

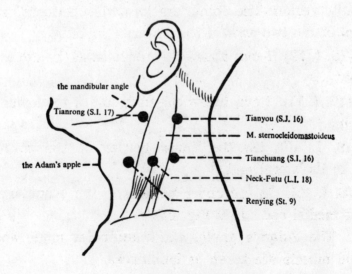

Fig. 26 Adam's Apple, Mandibular Angle and
Sternocleidomastoid Muscle as Landmarks

III. THE METHOD OF LOCATING POINTS OF THE THREE YANG CHANNELS OF FOOT

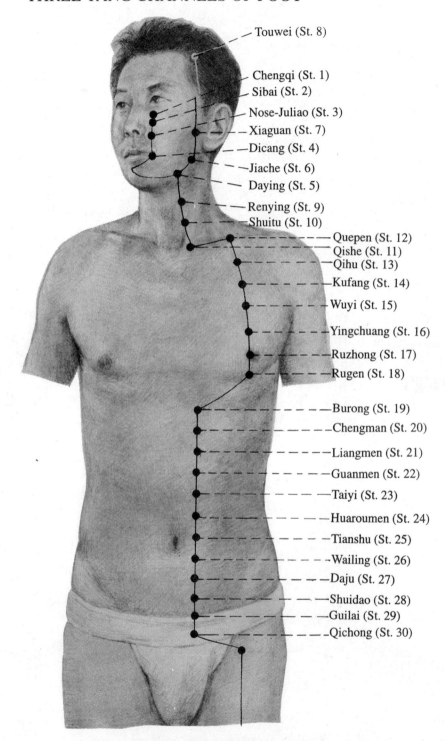

Touwei (St. 8)

Chengqi (St. 1)
Sibai (St. 2)
Nose-Juliao (St. 3)
Xiaguan (St. 7)
Dicang (St. 4)
Jiache (St. 6)
Daying (St. 5)
Renying (St. 9)
Shuitu (St. 10)
Quepen (St. 12)
Qishe (St. 11)
Qihu (St. 13)
Kufang (St. 14)
Wuyi (St. 15)
Yingchuang (St. 16)
Ruzhong (St. 17)
Rugen (St. 18)

Burong (St. 19)
Chengman (St. 20)
Liangmen (St. 21)
Guanmen (St. 22)
Taiyi (St. 23)
Huaroumen (St. 24)
Tianshu (St. 25)
Wailing (St. 26)
Daju (St. 27)
Shuidao (St. 28)
Guilai (St. 29)
Qichong (St. 30)

Fig. 27 The Stomach Channel of Foot-Yangming (1)

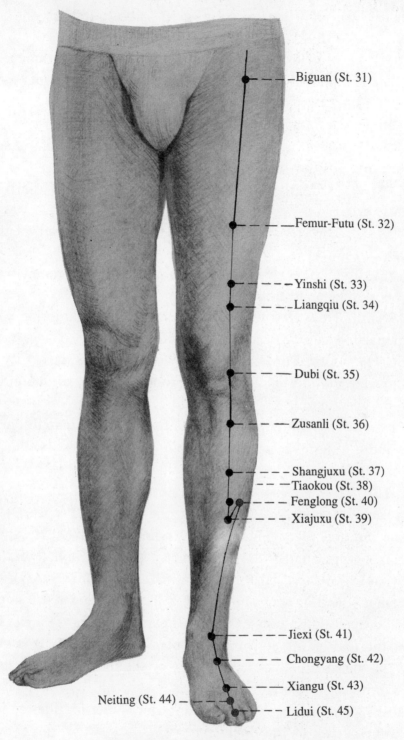

Biguan (St. 31)

Femur-Futu (St. 32)

Yinshi (St. 33)

Liangqiu (St. 34)

Dubi (St. 35)

Zusanli (St. 36)

Shangjuxu (St. 37)
Tiaokou (St. 38)
Fenglong (St. 40)
Xiajuxu (St. 39)

Jiexi (St. 41)

Chongyang (St. 42)

Xiangu (St. 43)

Neiting (St. 44)

Lidui (St. 45)

Fig. 27 The Stomach Channel of Foot-Yangming (2)

1. The Stomach Channel of Foot-Yangming

Chengqi (St. 1): 0.7 *cun* directly below the pupil at the infraorbital ridge.

Sibai (St. 2): 1 *cun* below the pupil, at the infraorbital foramen.

Nose-Juliao (St. 3): Directly below the pupil, at level of the lower border of ala nasi.

Dicang (St. 4): 0.4 *cun* lateral to the corner of mouth.

Daying (St. 5): 1.3 *cun* anterior and lower to the angle of mandible.

Jiache (St. 6): At the prominence of the masseter muscle.

Xiaguan (St. 7): Directly above Jiache (St. 6), on the lower border of the zygomatic arch.

Touwei (St. 8): Directly above the corner of the forehead, at the level of Shenting (D. 24).

Renying (St. 9): At the level of the Adam's apple, on the anterior border of sternocleidomastoid muscle.

Shuitu (St. 10): 1 *cun* below Renying (St. 9), on the anterior border of sternocleidomastoid muscle.

Qishe (St. 11): At the superior border of the sternal extremity of the clavicle, between the sternal head and clavicular head of the sternocleidomastoid muscle.

Quepen (St. 12): In the supraclavicular fossa, on the mammillary line.

Points on the chest: There are six points on the chest; Qihu (St. 13), Kufang (St. 14), Wuyi (St. 15), Yingchuang (St. 16), Ruzhong (St. 17), Rugen (St. 18). They are located 4 *cun* lateral to the middle line, one rib apart from each other. All of them are in the intercostal space.

Points on the abdomen: There are 12 points, Burong (St. 19), Chengman (St. 20), Liangmen (St. 21), Guanmen (St. 22), Taiyi (St. 23), Huaroumen (St. 24), Tianshu (St. 25), Wailing (St. 26), Daju (St. 27), Shuidao (St. 28), Guilai (St. 29), Qichong (St. 30). They are located 2 *cun* lateral to the middle line. Each point is 1 *cun* apart from the other. The distance from the end of the sternum to centre of the umbilicus is measured as 8 *cun*. The distance between the centre of the umbilicus and the upper border of symphysis pubis is 5 *cun*.

Biguan (St. 30): Directly below the anterior superior iliac spine, level with the lower border of the pubic symphysis.

The distance from the popliteal crease to the greater trochanter is measured as 19 *cun*.

Femur-Futu (St. 32): In the middle of the anterior aspect of the thigh, 6 *cun* above the knee.

Yinshi (St. 33): 3 *cun* above the knee.

Liangqiu (St. 34): 2 *cun* above the knee.

Both Yinshi and Liangqiu are on the line connecting Futu (St. 32) and supero-lateral border of the patella.

Dubi (St. 35): On the lateral foramen of the patella.

The method of locating Zusanli (St. 36), Shangjuxu (St. 37), Tiaokou (St. 38), Fenglong (St. 40) and Xiajuxu point.

The anterior tibial muscle appears protuberant when it is contraction. Zusanli (St. 36) is at the protuberance of the upper part of the muscle. Xiajuxu (St. 39) is at its lower end, Shangjuxu (St. 37) is at the mid-point of the line connecting Zusanli (St. 36) and Xiajuxu (St. 39). Shangjuxu (St. 37) is between Zusanli and Xiajuxu (St. 39). Tiaokou (St. 38) is 1 *cun* above Xiajuxu (St. 39). Fenglong (St. 40) is lateral to Tiaokou (St. 39), on the border of the muscle.

Jiexi (St. 41): At the level of the tip of the external malleolus, between the two tendons on the anterior aspect of the ankle joint (i.e. between the tendons of m. extensor digitorum longus and hallucis longus).

Chongyang (St. 42): 1.3 *cun* below Jiexi (St. 41), on the pulse of the dorsal artery.

Xiangu (St. 43) and Neiting (St. 44): Both are between the 2nd and the 3rd metatarsophalangeal joints. Xiangu (St. 43) is posterior to the joints. Neiting (St. 44) is anterior to the joint.

Lidui (St. 45): At the outer corner of the nail of the 2nd toe.

How to locate the points of this channel?

You may find them the upper, middle and lower parts and the border of the anterior tibial muscles.

Zusanli (St. 36) is at the protuberance of the upper part of the muscle. Xiajuxu (St. 39) is at its lower end. Shangjuxu (St. 37) is in the middle of the muscle. Tiaokou (St. 38) is 1 *cun* above Xiajuxu (St. 39). Fenglong (St. 40) is lateral to Tiaokou (St. 38), on the border of the muscle.

2. The Urinary Bladder Channel of Foot-Taiyang

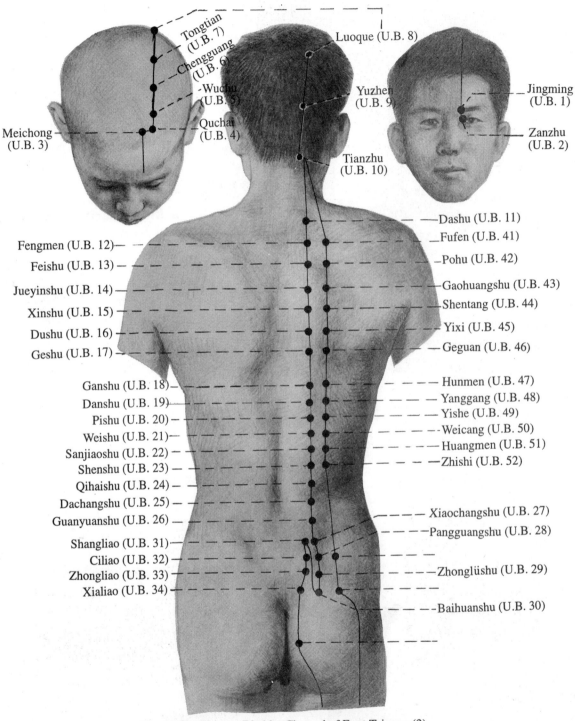

Tongtian (U.B. 7)
Chengguang (U.B. 6)
Wuchu (U.B. 5)
Quchai (U.B. 4)
Meichong (U.B. 3)
Luoque (U.B. 8)
Yuzhen (U.B. 9)
Tianzhu (U.B. 10)
Jingming (U.B. 1)
Zanzhu (U.B. 2)

Fengmen (U.B. 12)—
Feishu (U.B. 13) —
Jueyinshu (U.B. 14) —
Xinshu (U.B. 15) —
Dushu (U.B. 16) —
Geshu (U.B. 17) —
Ganshu (U.B. 18)—
Danshu (U.B. 19)—
Pishu (U.B. 20) —
Weishu (U.B. 21)—
Sanjiaoshu (U.B. 22) —
Shenshu (U.B. 23) —
Qihaishu (U.B. 24) —
Dachangshu (U.B. 25) —
Guanyuanshu (U.B. 26) —
Shangliao (U.B. 31)—
Ciliao (U.B. 32) —
Zhongliao (U.B. 33)—
Xialiao (U.B. 34)—

Dashu (U.B. 11)
Fufen (U.B. 41)
Pohu (U.B. 42)
Gaohuangshu (U.B. 43)
Shentang (U.B. 44)
Yixi (U.B. 45)
Geguan (U.B. 46)
Hunmen (U.B. 47)
Yanggang (U.B. 48)
Yishe (U.B. 49)
Weicang (U.B. 50)
Huangmen (U.B. 51)
Zhishi (U.B. 52)
Xiaochangshu (U.B. 27)
Pangguangshu (U.B. 28)
Zhonglüshu (U.B. 29)
Baihuanshu (U.B. 30)

Fig. 28 The Urinary Bladder Channel of Foot-Taiyang (2)

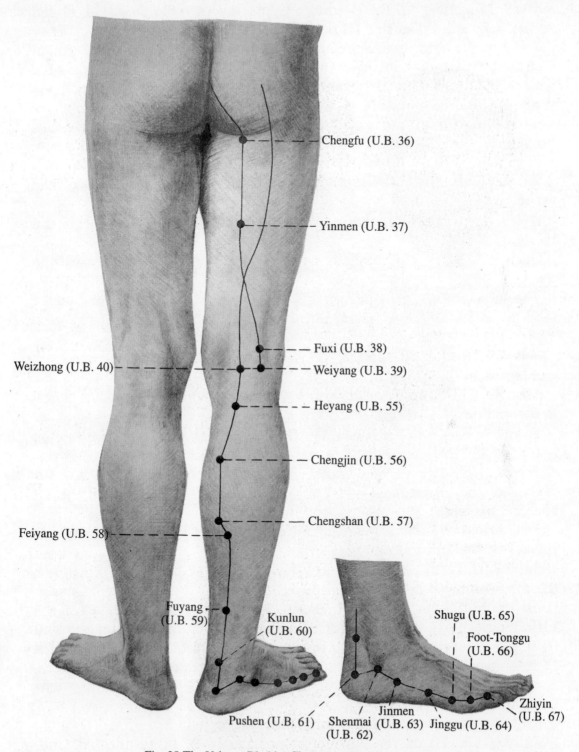

Fig. 28 The Urinary Bladder Channel of Foot-Taiyang (2)

The Urinary Bladder Channel of Foot-Taiyang: It starts at the inner canthus (Jingming, U.B. 1) and ascends through the forehead to the vertex. At point Tianzhu (U.B. 10), it separates into two lines. They descend to the back, lumbar region and the posterior aspect of the thigh, and combine into one in the popliteal fossa. Then it again descends passing the posterior part of the external malleolus, and ending at the small toe (Zhiyin, U.B. 67).

From the anterior hairline to the posterior hairline, the distance is measured as 12 *cun*. The distance between the two mastoid processes is 9 *cun*.

Jingming (U.B. 1): 0.1 *cun* superior to the inner canthus.

Zanzhu (U.B. 2): On the supraorbital notch, at the medial end of the eyebrow.

Meichong (U.B. 3): Directly above Zanzhu (U.B. 2), 0.5 *cun* within the hairline.

Quchai (U.B. 4): 1.5 *cun* lateral to the midline, 0.5 *cun* within the hairline.

Wuchu (U.B. 5), Chengguang (U.B. 6), Tongtian (U.B. 7), and Luoque (U.B. 8): All are 1.5 *cun* lateral to the midline, 1.5 *cun* apart from each other.

Yuzhen (U.B. 9): At superior border of the occipital protuberance, 1.3 *cun* lateral to the midline.

Tianzhu (U.B. 10): 0.5 *cun* within the posterior hairline, 1.3 *cun* lateral to the midline.

Points on back and lumbar region: The first line between every vertebra is 1.5 *cun* and the second line is 3 *cun* lateral to the midline of the back.

Dazhu (U.B. 11): 1.5 *cun* lateral to the lower border of the spinous process of the 1st thoracic vertebra (at the level of space between the 1st and 2nd vertebra).

Fengmen (U.B. 12): 1.5 *cun* lateral to the lower border of the spinous process of the 2nd thoracic vertebra.

Feishu (U.B. 13) on the 3rd, Jueyinshu (U.B. 14) on the 4th, Xinshu on the 5th, Dushu (U.B. 16) on the 6th, Geshu (U.B. 17) on the 7th, Ganshu (U.B. 18) on the 9th, Danshu (U.B. 19) on the 10th, Pishu (U.B. 20) on the 11th, Weishu (U.B. 21) on the 12th, Sanjiaoshu (U.B. 22) the 13th, Shenshu (U.B. 23) the 14th, Qihaishu (U.B. 24) the 15th, Dachangshu (U.B. 25) the 16th, Guanyuanshu (U.B. 26) the 17th, Xiaochangshu (U.B. 27) the 18th, Pangguangshu (U.B. 28) the 19th, Zhonglushu (U.B. 29) the 20th, Baihuanshu (U.B. 30) the 21st.

On the second line are following points:

Fufen (U.B. 41) on the 2nd vertebra, Pohu (U.B. 42) on the 3rd, Gaohuangshu (U.B. 43) on the 4th, Shentang (U.B. 44) on the 5th, Yixi (U.B. 45) on the 6th, Geguan (U.B. 46) on the 7th, Hunmen (U.B. 47) on the 9th,

Yanggang (U.B. 48) on the 10th, Yishe (U.B. 49) on the 11th, Weicang (U.B. 50) on the 12th, Huangmen (U.B. 51) on the 13th, Zhishi (U.B. 52) on the 14th, Baohuang (U.B. 53) on the 19th, Zhibian (U.B. 54) on the 21st.

Shangliao, Ciliao, Zhongliao and Xialiao points: (See Fig. 29)

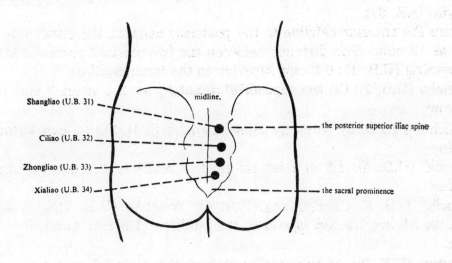

Fig. 29 Eight Liaos

Shangliao (U.B. 31) midway between the posterior superior iliac spine and the dorsal midline. Xialiao (U.B. 34) the depression which is superior and exterior to the sacral prominence. Divide the distance from Shangliao (U.B. 31) to Xialiao (U.B. 34) into 3 equal parts with two dots, the 1st one is the locations of Ciliao (U.B. 32) and the second one being Zhongliao (U.B. 33).

Huiyang (U.B. 35): On either side of the tip of the coccyx, 0.5 *cun* lateral to the midline.

Chengfu (U.B. 36): At the midpoint of the gluteal fold. The distance from Chengfu (U.B. 36) to the popliteal crease is measured as 14 *cun*. Yinmen (U.B. 37) is 6 *cun* below Chengfu (U.B. 36), on the middle of the posterior aspect of the thigh.

Fuxi (U.B. 38) and Weiyang (U.B. 39): Both the points are on the medial side of the tendon of m. biceps femoris. Weiyang (U.B. 39) is at the level of Weizhong (U.B. 40) and Fuxi (U.B. 38) is 1 *cun* above Weiyang (U.B. 39).

Weizhong (U.B. 40) is in the midpoint of the transverse crease of the popliteal fossa, between the tendons of m. biceps femoris and s. semitendinosus.

The distance between the popliteal crease and the tip of the lateral malleolus is measured as 16 *cun*.

How to locate Heyang (U.B. 55), Chengjin (U.B. 56), Chengshan (U.B. 57) and Feiyang (U.B. 58)?

Some points are named by ancient doctors according to anatomical landmarks. Heyang (U.B. 55) is where the two heads of the gastrocnemius muscle meet, and Chengshan (U.B. 57) is where the two heads separate, like a hill. Chengjin (U.B. 56) is at the midpoint between Heyang (U.B. 55) and Chengshan (U.B. 57). Feiyang (U.B. 58) 1 *cun* exterior and inferior to Chengshan (U.B. 57), is at the border of the muscle.

How to locate Fuyang (U.B. 59), Kunlun (U.B. 60) and Pushen (U.B. 61)?

Kunlun (U.B. 60) is between the tip of the external malleolus and posterior border of the tendocalcaneus. Fuyang (U.B. 59) is 3 *cun* directly above Kunlun (U.B. 60), Pushen (U.B. 61) is 2 *cun* directly below Kunlun (U.B. 60).

Shenmai (U.B. 62): 0.5 *cun* below the lower border of the external malleolus, directly below its tip.

Jinmen (U.B. 63): Directly below the anterior border of the external malleolus, in the depression below the cuboid bone.

Jinggu (U.B. 64): Anterior and inferior to the tuberosity of the 5th metatarsal bone, at the external aspect of the foot.

Shugu (U.B. 66): Anterior and external to the joint.

Zhiyin (U.B. 67): Posterior to the lateral corner of the nail at the small toe.

How to locate the points of this channel?

Heyang (U.B. 55), Chengjin (U.B. 56), Chengshan (U.B. 57) and Feiyang (U.B. 58) are all located according to the anatomical feature of m. gastrocuomius.

3. The Gall Bladder Channel Of Foot Shaoyang

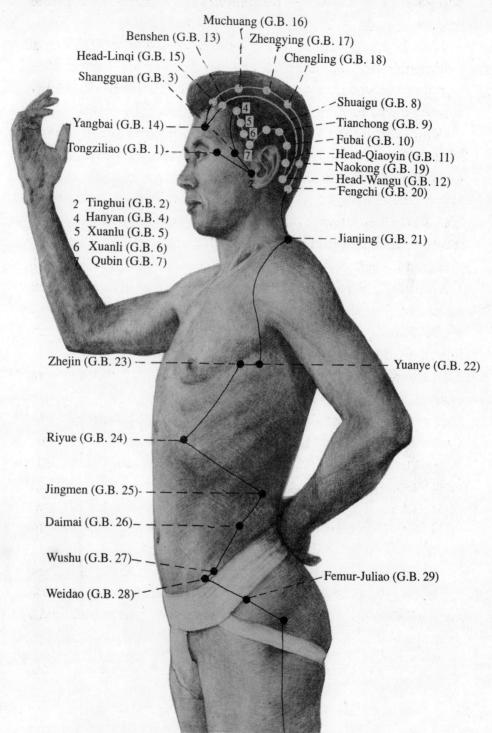

Muchuang (G.B. 16)
Benshen (G.B. 13)
Zhengying (G.B. 17)
Head-Linqi (G.B. 15)
Chengling (G.B. 18)
Shangguan (G.B. 3)
Shuaigu (G.B. 8)
Yangbai (G.B. 14) —
Tianchong (G.B. 9)
Fubai (G.B. 10)
Tongziliao (G.B. 1) -
Head-Qiaoyin (G.B. 11)
Naokong (G.B. 19)
Head-Wangu (G.B. 12)
Fengchi (G.B. 20)

2 Tinghui (G.B. 2)
4 Hanyan (G.B. 4)
5 Xuanlu (G.B. 5)
6 Xuanli (G.B. 6)
7 Qubin (G.B. 7)

Jianjing (G.B. 21)

Zhejin (G.B. 23) -
Yuanye (G.B. 22)

Riyue (G.B. 24) -

Jingmen (G.B. 25)-

Daimai (G.B. 26)-

Wushu (G.B. 27)-

Femur-Juliao (G.B. 29)
Weidao (G.B. 28)-

Fig. 30 The Gall Bladder Channel Of Foot-Shaoyang (1)

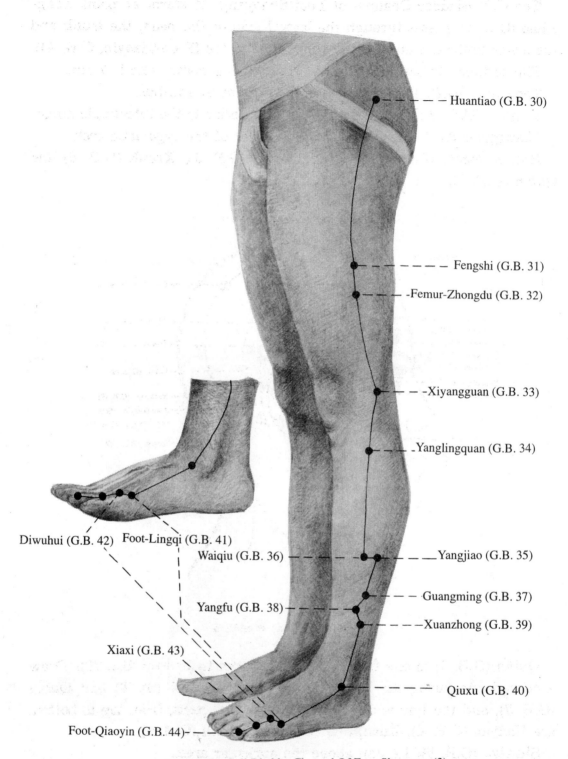

Huantiao (G.B. 30)

Fengshi (G.B. 31)

-Femur-Zhongdu (G.B. 32)

-Xiyangguan (G.B. 33)

-Yanglingquan (G.B. 34)

Diwuhui (G.B. 42)   Foot-Lingqi (G.B. 41)

Waiqiu (G.B. 36)   Yangjiao (G.B. 35)

Guangming (G.B. 37)

Yangfu (G.B. 38)

Xuanzhong (G.B. 39)

Xiaxi (G.B. 43)

Qiuxu (G.B. 40)

Foot-Qiaoyin (G.B. 44)

Fig. 30 The Gall Bladder Channel Of Foot-Shaoyang (2)

The Gall Bladder Channel of Foot-Shaoyang: It starts at point Tong-ziliao (G.B. 1), passes through the lateral side of the head, the trunk and the lower limb, and ends at the tip of the 4th toe (Foot-Qiaoyin, G.B. 44).

The distance between the tip of the two zygomatic bone is 7 *cun*.

Tongziliao (G.B. 1): 0.5 *cun* lateral to the outer canthus.

Tinghui (G.B. 2): In the depression of anterior to the intertragic notch.

Shangguan (G.B. 3): On the upper border of the zygomatic arch.

How to locate Hanyan (G.B. 4), Xuanlu (G.B. 5), Xuanli (G.B. 6) and Qubin (G.B. 7)?

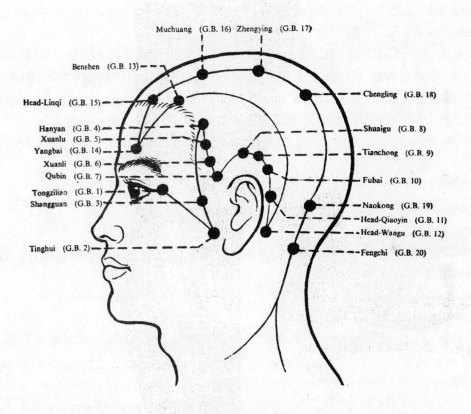

Fig. 31 Points of G.B. Channel on Head

Qubin (G.B. 7) is one finger-breadth anterior to Jiaosun (S.J. 20). Draw a curved line (along the hairline) connecting Touwei (St. 8) and Qubin (G.B. 7), and the line is divided into four equal parts, from top to bottom are Hanyan (G.B. 4), Xuanlu (G.B. 5) and Xuanli (G.B. 6).

Shuaigu (G.B. 8): 1.4 *cun* above the auricular apex.

Tianchong (G.B. 9): 1.5 *cun* posterior and inferior to Shuaigu (G.B. 8).

Fubai (G.B. 10): 1 *cun* inferior and posterior to Tianchong (G.B. 9).

Head-Qiaoyin (G.B. 11): On the posterior and superior aspect of the mastoid process.

Head-Wangu (G.B. 12): On the posterior and inferior aspect of the mastoid process.

Benshen (G.B. 13): 0.5 *cun* within the hairline, 3 *cun* lateral to the midline of the head.

Yangbai (G.B. 14): 1 *cun* above the midpoint of the eyebrow.

Head-Linqi (G.B. 15): 0.5 *cun* within the hairline, at the midway between the Touwei (St. 8) and the midline of the head.

How to locate Muchuang (G.B. 16), Zhengying (G.B. 17) and Chengling (G.B. 18)?

Muchuang (G.B. 16) is 1.5 *cun* posterior to Head-Linqi (G.B. 15).

Both Zhengying (G.B. 17) and Chengling (G.B. 18) are posterior to Muchuang (G.B. 16), 1.5 *cun* apart from each other, the three points are 2.25 *cun* lateral to the midline. Naokong (G.B. 19) is midway between the superior border of the occipital protuberance and the superior border of the mastoid.

Fengchi (G.B. 20) at the midpoint between the inferior border of the mastoid process and Fengfu (Du. 16) is 1 *cun* above the posterior hairline, at the midline.

Jianjing (G.B. 21): Between the midpoint of the clavicle and the superior border of the scapula.

Yuanye (G.B. 22): 3 *cun* directly below the axillary centre, in the 4th intercostal space.

Zhejin (G.B. 23): 1 *cun* anterior to Yuanye (G.B. 22) in the 4th intercostal space.

Riyue (G.B. 24): 3 ribs below the nipple, in the 7th intercosted space.

Jingmen (G.B. 25): On the free end of the 12th rib.

Daimai (G.B. 26): Directly below the free end of the 11th rib, at the level of the umbillicus.

Wushu (G.B. 27): 0.5 *cun* in front of the anterior superior iliac spine.

Weidao (G.B. 28): 0.5 *cun* anterior and inferior to Wushu (G.B. 27).

Juliao (G.B. 29): Midway between the anterior superior iliac spine and the greater trachanter.

Huantiao (G.B. 30): Midway between the anterior superior border of the greater trochanter and the hiatus of the sacrum.

Fengshi (G.B. 31): In the centre of the lateral side of the thigh, 7 *cun* above the transverse popliteal crease.

Zhongdu (G.B. 32): 2 *cun* below Fengshi (G.B. 31).

Knee-Yangguan (G.B. 33): In the depression superior to the lateral epicondyle of the femur, in front of the tendon of m. biceps femoris.

Yanglingquan (G.B. 34): In the depression anterior and inferior to the small head of the fibula.

Waiqiu (G.B. 36) and Yangjiao (G.B. 35) are 7 *cun* above the external malleolus. Waiqiu (G.B. 36) is on the anterior border of the fibula, and Yangjiao (G.B. 35) is on the posterior border of the fibula.

Guangming (G.B. 37): 5 *cun* above the tip of the external malleolus, on the posterior border of the fibula.

Yangfu (G.B. 38): 4 *cun* above the tip of the external malleolus, on the anterior border of the fibula.

Xuanzhong (G.B. 39): 3 *cun* above the tip of the external malleolus, on the posterior border of the fibula.

Qiuxu (G.B. 40): In the depression anterior and inferior to the external mallealus.

Foot-Lingqi (G.B. 41): Posterior to the tendon of m. extensor digiti minimi pedis, in front of the junction of the 4th and 5th metatarsal bones.

Diwuhui (G.B. 42): On cleft between the 4th and 5th metatarsal bones, posterior to the metatarsophalangeal joint.

Xiaxi (G.B. 43): On the cleft between the 4th and 5th metatarsal bones, anterior to the metatorsophalangeal joint.

Foot-Qiaoying (G.B. 44): Posterior to the lateral corner of the nail at the 4th toe.

How to locate the points of this channel?

The anterior and the posterior border of the fibula.

Yanglingquan (G.B. 34), Waiqiu (G.B. 36) and Yangfu (G.B. 38) are on the anterior border of the fibula, and Yangjiao (G.B. 35), Guangming (G.B. 37) and Xuanzhong (G.B. 39) are on the posterior border of the fibula.

4. The Summing-up of the Three Yang Channels of Foot According-ing to the Different Parts of the Body

1. Tips of the Toe:

Lidui (St. 45), Foot-Qiaoyin (G.B. 44) and Zhiyin (U.B. 67) are at the lateral corners of the root of nails. (Fig. 32)

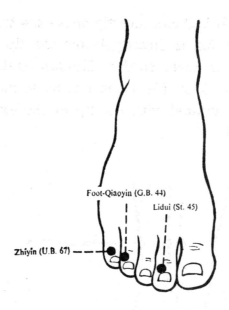

Foot-Qiaoyin (G.B. 44)

Lidui (St. 45)

Zhiyin (U.B. 67)

Fig. 32 Points at Nail Corners

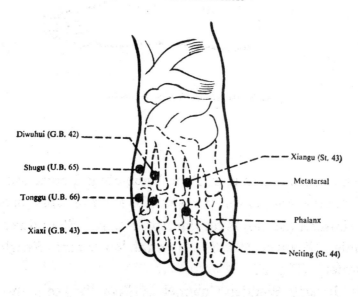

Diwuhui (G.B. 42)

Shugu (U.B. 65)

Tonggu (U.B. 66)

Xiaxi (G.B. 43)

Xiangu (St. 43)

Metatarsal

Phalanx

Neiting (St. 44)

Fig. 33 Points Anterior or Posterior to Metatarsophalangeal Joints

2.   Metatarsus: Points are located anteriorly or posteriorly to metatarsophalangeal joints: Neiting (St. 44) and Xiangu (St. 43) of the Stomach Channel, Xiaxi (G.B. 43) and Diwuhui (G.B. 42) of the Gall Bladder Channel, and Tonggu (U.B. 66) and Shugu (U.B. 65) of the Urinary Bladder.

3. Xuanzhong (G.B. 39) is 3 *cun* directly above the tip of the external malleolus. Shenmai (U.B. 62) is directly below the tip of the external malleolus, 0.5 *cun* below its lower border. Kunlun (U.B. 60) is posterior to the external malleolus. Jiexi (St. 41) is anterior to the external malleolus. All these points are located with the tip of the external malleolus as the landmark. (Fig. 34)

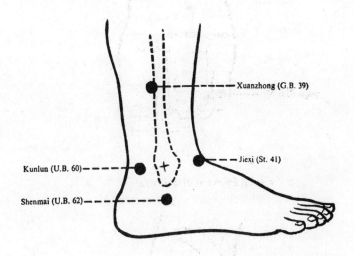

Fig. 34 Points Around Tip of Malleolus

4. Leg:

(1) The Stomach Channel of Foot Yangming: Points are located on the upper, middle and lower parts of the anterior tibial muscle and on its border. Zusanli (St. 36) is on the upper part. Shangjuxu (St. 37) is in the middle. Xiajuxu (St. 39) is on the lower part. Fenglong (St. 40) is on its border. (Fig. 35)

(2) The Urinary Bladder Channel of Foot Taiyang: the gastrocnemius muscle is taken as the landmark.

Heyang (U.B. 55) is located where the two heads of the muscle meet.

Chengshan (U.B. 57) is located where the two heads of the muscle separate.

Chengjin (U.B. 56) is between Heyang (U.B. 55) and Chengshan (U.B. 57).

Feiyang (U.B. 58) is on the border of the gastrocnemius. 1 *cun* lateral and inferior to Chengshan (U.B. 57). (Fig. 36)

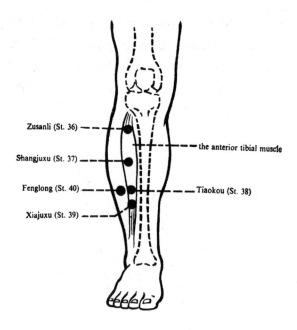

Zusanli (St. 36)

Shangjuxu (St. 37)

Fenglong (St. 40)

Xiajuxu (St. 39)

the anterior tibial muscle

Tiaokou (St. 38)

Fig. 35 Points on and near Anterior Tibial Muscle

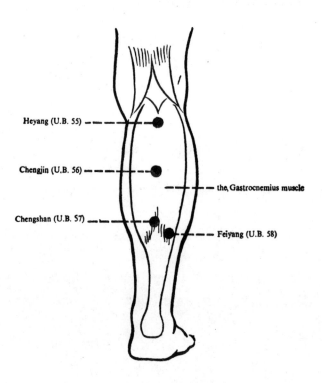

Heyang (U.B. 55)

Chengjin (U.B. 56)

Chengshan (U.B. 57)

the Gastrocnemius muscle

Feiyang (U.B. 58)

Fig. 36 Points on Gastrocnemius Muscle

(3) The Gall Bladder Channel of Foot Shaoyang: Points are anterior or posterior to the fibula. Yanglingquan (G.B. 34), Waiqiu (G.B. 36) and Yangfu (G.B. 38) are on the anterior border of the fibula. Yangjiao (G.B. 35), Guangming (G.B. 37) and Xuanzhong (G.B. 39) are on the posterior border of the fibula. (Fig. 37)

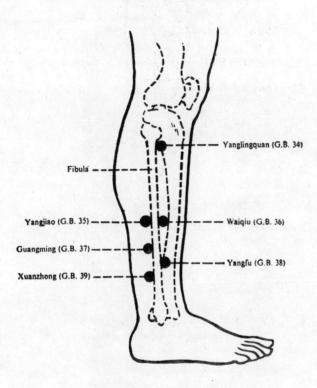

Fig. 37 Points Anterior or Posterior to Fibula

IV. THE METHOD OF LOCATING POINTS ON THE THREE YIN CHANNELS OF FOOT

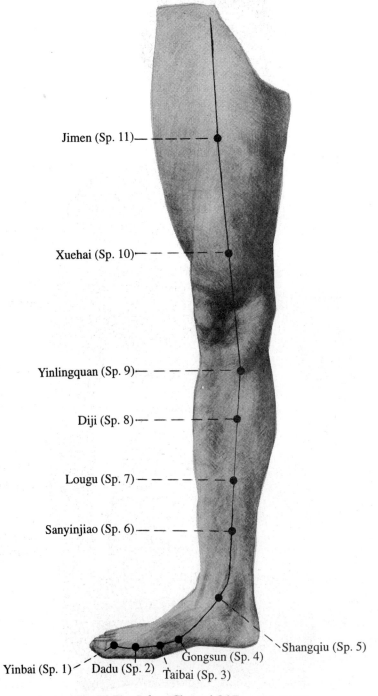

Fig. 38 The Spleen Channel Of Foot-Taiyin (1)

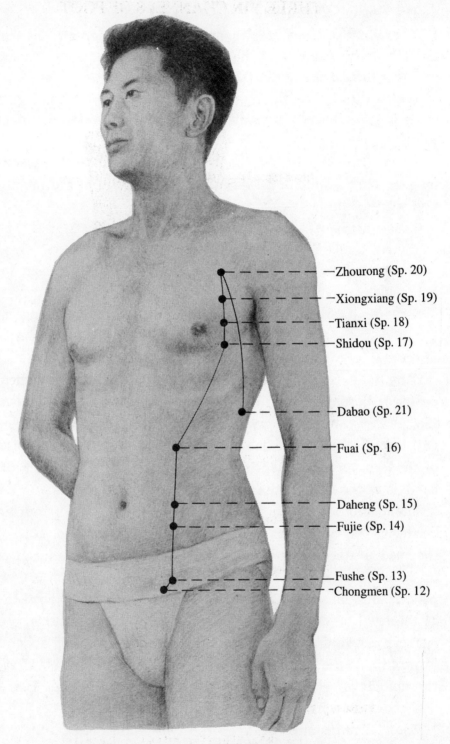

—Zhourong (Sp. 20)

—Xiongxiang (Sp. 19)

—Tianxi (Sp. 18)

—Shidou (Sp. 17)

—Dabao (Sp. 21)

—Fuai (Sp. 16)

—Daheng (Sp. 15)

—Fujie (Sp. 14)

—Fushe (Sp. 13)
—Chongmen (Sp. 12)

Fig. 38 The Spleen Channel Of Foot-Taiyin (2)

1. The Spleen Channel of Foot-Taiyin

The Spleen Channel of Foot-Taiyin:

It originates from the medial side of the great toe, runs along the anterior medial aspect of the lower limb and up to the abdomen and chest, and ends below the axilla (Dabao, Sp. 21).

Yinbai (Sp. 1): At the medial corner of root of the nail in the great toe.

Dadu (Sp. 2): On the medial and distal to the 1st metatarsophalangeal joint.

Taibai (Sp. 3): On the medial and proximal to the 1st metatarsophalangeal joint. Tabai and Dadu (Sp. 2) points are at the junction of the red and white skin.

Gongsun (Sp. 4): 1 *cun* posterior to Taibai (Sp. 3), also at the junction of the red and white skin.

Shangqiu (Sp. 5): In the depression distal and inferior to the medial malleolus.

Sanyinjiao (Sp. 6), Lougu (Sp. 7), Diji (Sp. 8) and Yinlingquan (Sp. 9):

The distance from the tip of the medial malleolus to the lower border of the medial condyle of the tibia is measured as 13 *cun*.

Sanyinjiao (Sp. 6) is 3 *cun* above the tip of the medial malleolus, near the posterior border of the tibia. Lougu (Sp. 7) is 3 *cun* above Sanyinjiao (Sp. 6). Diji (Sp. 8) is 4 *cun* above Lougu (Sp. 7). Both Lougu (Sp. 7) and Diji (Sp. 8) are located one finger-breadth lateral to the posterior border of the tibia. Yinlingquan (Sp. 9) is on the inferior border of the medial condyle of the tibia at the posterior border of the tibia.

The distance between the medial epicondyle of the femur and the upper border of the symphysis pubis is 18 *cun*. Xuehai (Sp. 10) is 2 *cun* above the medial epicondyle of the femur, at the protuberance of the m. vastus medialis. Jimen (Sp. 11) is 6 *cun* above Xuehai (Sp. 10), at the ending part of this muscle. Chongmen (Sp. 12) is 3.5 *cun* lateral to the midline, at the level of the superior border of the symphisis pubis. Fushe (Sp. 13) is 1 *cun* above Chongmen (Sp. 12), 4 *cun* lateral to the abdominal midline. Fujie (Sp. 14) is 1.3 *cun* below Daheng (Sp. 15) which is at the level of the umbilicus, 4 *cun* lateral to the abdominal midline. Fuai (Sp. 16) is 3 *cun* above Daheng (Sp. 15).

Chest: The distance between the two nipples is 8 *cun*.

Shidou (Sp. 17): On the chest, in the 5th intercostal space, 6 *cun* lateral to the midline.

Tianxi (Sp. 18): In the 4th intercostal space, 6 *cun* lateral to the midline.

Xiongxiang (Sp. 19): In the 3rd intercostal space, 6 *cun* lateral to the midline.

Zhourong (Sp. 20): In the 2nd intercostal space, 6 *cun* lateral to the midline.

Dabao (Sp. 21): In the 6th intercostal space 6 *cun* directly below the centre of axilla.

How to locate the points of this channel?

Find them at border of the bone, or measure with one finger breadth.

Sanyinjiao (Sp. 6) and Yinlingquan (Sp. 9) are on the posterior border of the tibia. Lougu (Sp. 7) and Diji (Sp. 8) are one finger-breadth posterior to the tibial border.

2. The Kidney Channel Of Foot-Shaoyin

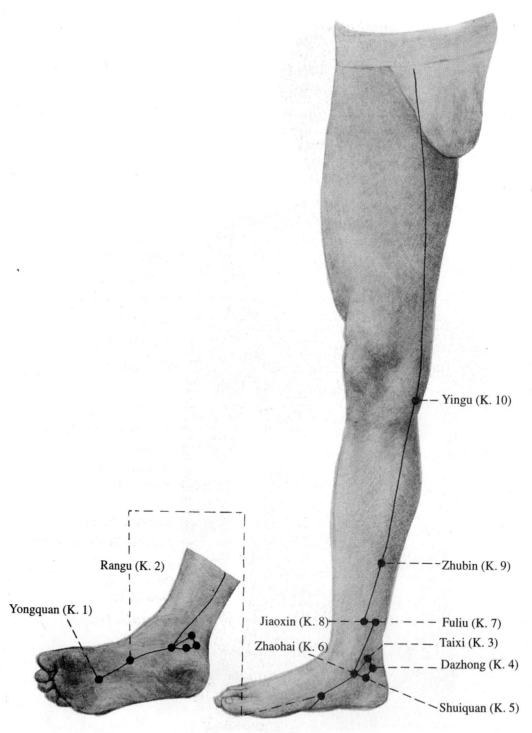

Yingu (K. 10)

Zhubin (K. 9)

Rangu (K. 2)

Yongquan (K. 1)

Jiaoxin (K. 8)

Fuliu (K. 7)

Zhaohai (K. 6)

Taixi (K. 3)

Dazhong (K. 4)

Shuiquan (K. 5)

Fig. 39 The Kidney Channel Of Foot-Shaoyin (1)

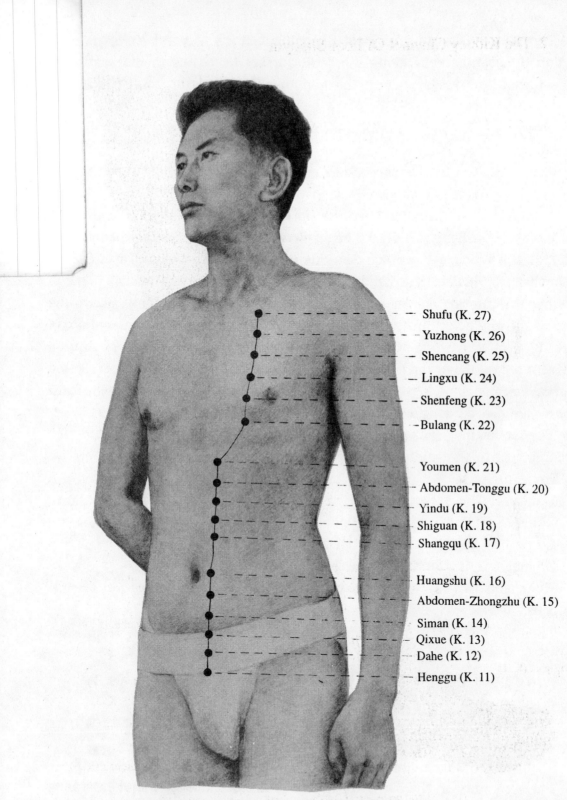

—— Shufu (K. 27)
—— Yuzhong (K. 26)
—— Shencang (K. 25)
—— Lingxu (K. 24)
—— Shenfeng (K. 23)
——Bulang (K. 22)

—— Youmen (K. 21)
—— Abdomen-Tonggu (K. 20)
—— Yindu (K. 19)
—— Shiguan (K. 18)
—— Shangqu (K. 17)

—— Huangshu (K. 16)
—— Abdomen-Zhongzhu (K. 15)
—— Siman (K. 14)
—— Qixue (K. 13)
—— Dahe (K. 12)
—— Henggu (K. 11)

Fig. 39 The Kidney Channel Of Foot-Shaoyin (2)

The Kidney Channel of Foot-Shaoyin: It starts at point Yongquan (K. 1) on the sole, ascends along the posterior border of the medial aspect of the lower limb, passes along the abdomen and ends at point Shufu (K. 27) on the chest.

Yongquan (K. 1): In the depression which is at the junction of the anterior and middle third of the sole.

Rangu (K. 2): In the depression on anterior and inferior to the tuberosity of the navicular bone.

Taixi (K. 3): Midway between the tip of the medial malleolus and tendo calcaneus. Dazhong (K. 4): 0.5 cun below Taixi (K. 3), on the medial border of the tendo calcaneus. Shuiquan (K. 5): 1 cun below Taixi (K. 3). Zhaohai (K. 6): Directly below the tip of the medial malleolus, 0.4 cun below the inferior border of the malleolus. Fuliu (K. 7): 2 cun above the tip of the malleolus, on the anterior border of the tendo calcaneus. Jiaoxin (K. 8): Between the posterior border of the tibia and Fuliu (K. 7). Zhubin (K. 9): 5 cun above the tip of the malleolus, on the anterior border of the tendo calcaneus. Yingu (K. 10): On the medial side of the popliteal fossa between the tendons of m. semitendinosus and semimembranosus.

The following six points on the lower abdomen are located 0.5 cun lateral to the midline and are 1 cun apart from each other.

Henggu (K. 11): On the superior border of the public symphysis.

Dahe (K. 12): 1 cun above Henggu (K. 11).

Qixue (K. 13): 1 cun above Dahe (K. 12).

Siman (K. 14): 1 cun above Qixue (K. 13).

Zhongzhu (K. 15): 1 cun above Siman (K. 14).

Huangshu (K. 16): 1 cun above Zhongzhu (K. 15), at the level of umbilicus.

Then the five points on the upper abdomen are 1 cun apart from each other and also 0.5 cun lateral to the abdominal midline.

Shangqu (K. 17): 2 cun above umbilicus, 0.5 cun lateral to the midline.

Shiguan (K. 18): 1 cun directly above Shangqu (K. 17).

Yindu (K. 19): 1 cun directly above Shiguan (K. 18).

Tonggu (K. 20): 1 cun directly above Yindu (K. 19).

Youmen (K. 21): 1 cun directly above Tonggu (K. 20).

The six points on the chest are in the intercostal space, 2 cun lateral to the abdominal midline, one rib apart from each other.

Bulang (K. 22): In the 5th intercostal space.

Shenfeng (K. 23): In the 4th intercostal space.

Lingxu (K. 24): In the 3rd intercostal space.

Shencang (K. 25): In the 2nd intercostal space.

Yuzhong (K. 26): In the 1st intercostal space.

Shufu (K. 27): At the lower border of the clavicle.

How to locate the points of this channel?

They are on the border of the tendon.

Dazhong (K. 4), Fuliu (K. 7) and Zhubin (K. 9) are all located near the anterior border of the tendo calcaneus.

3. The Liver Channel Of Foot-Jueyin

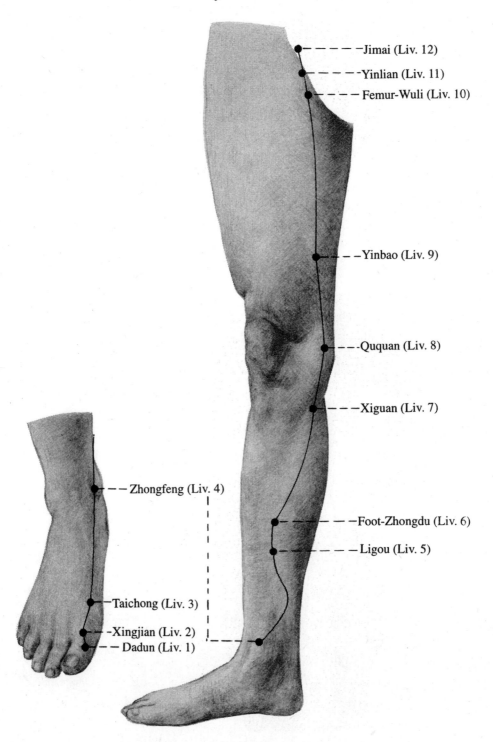

Jimai (Liv. 12)

Yinlian (Liv. 11)

Femur-Wuli (Liv. 10)

Yinbao (Liv. 9)

Ququan (Liv. 8)

Xiguan (Liv. 7)

Zhongfeng (Liv. 4)

Foot-Zhongdu (Liv. 6)

Ligou (Liv. 5)

Taichong (Liv. 3)

Xingjian (Liv. 2)

Dadun (Liv. 1)

Fig. 40 The Liver Channel Of Foot-Jueyin (1)

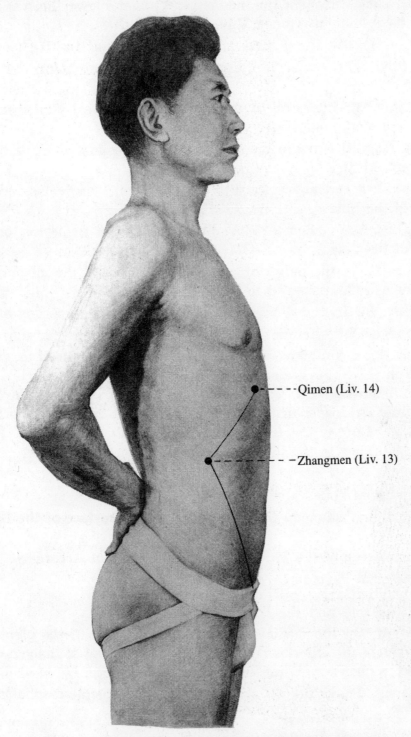

- - - Qimen (Liv. 14)

- - - Zhangmen (Liv. 13)

Fig. 40 The Liver Channel Of Foot-Jueyin (2)

The Liver Channel of Foot-Jueyin: It starts at point Dadun (Liv. 1) on the great toe, passes through the medial aspect of the lower limb and abdomen and ends at point Qimen (Liv. 14) on the chest.

Dadun (Liv. 1): At the lateral ¼ of the nail root of the big toe.

Xingjian (Liv. 2): Anterior to the metatarsophalangeal joint, between the first and second toe.

Taichong (Liv. 3): Posterior to the metatarsophalangeal joint, between the 1st and 2nd metatarsal bone.

Zhongfeng (Liv. 4): On the medial side of the tendon of m. extensor hallucis, level with the tip of the medial malleolus.

Ligou (Liv. 5): 5 *cun* above the tip of the medial malleolus, on the medial side of the tibia.

Zhongdu (Liv. 6): 7 *cun* above the tip of the medial malleolus, on the medial side of the tibia.

Xiguan (Liv. 7): In the posterior and inferior aspect of the medial condyle of the tibia, 1 *cun* posterior to Yinlingquan (Sp. 9).

Ququan (Liv. 8): In the depression between the upper border of the medial epicondyle of the femur and the tendon of m. semimembranosus.

Yinbao (Liv. 9): 4 *cun* above Ququan (Liv. 8), on the border of m. vastus medialis. Wuli (Liv. 10): 2 *cun* below Jimai (Liv. 12). Yinlian (Liv. 11): 1 *cun* below Jimai (Liv. 12). Jimai (Liv. 12): 2.5 *cun* lateral to the midpoint of the inferior border of the pubic symphysis, at the inguinal groove. Zhangmen (Liv. 13): At the free end of the 11th rib. Qimen (Liv. 14): 2 ribs below the nipple, in the intercostal space.

How to locate the points of this channel?

Contact the tibial bone.

Ligou (Liv. 5) and Zhongdu (Liv. 6) on the medial surface of the tibia.

4. The Summing-up of the Three Yin Channels of Foot According to Different Parts of the body

1. Foot: The sole and the corner of the nail root.

Yinbai (Sp. 1): On the medial corner of the nail root of the great toe. Dadun (Liv. 1): On the exterior one fourth of the nail root of the great toe. (See Fig. 41) (1), (2).

2. Metatarsus: Points are distal or Proximal the metatarsophalangeal joints.

The spleen channel: Dadu (Sp. 2), Taibai (Sp. 3).

The liver channel: Xingjian (Liv. 2), Taichong (Liv. 3). These points are distal or proximal to the joints. (See Fig. 42)

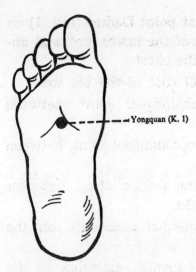

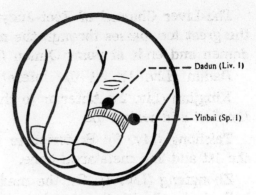

Fig. 41(2) Nail Corner

Fig. 41(1) Sole

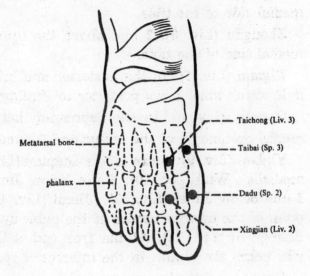

Fig. 42(1) Points Distal and Proximal to Metatarsophalangeal Joints

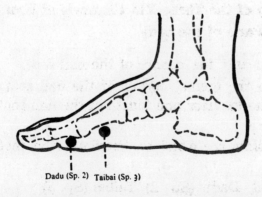

Fig. 42(2) Points Distal and Proximal to Metatarsophalangeal Joints

Superior, inferior, anterior and posterior to the tip of the malleolus.

3. Malleolus: Points are located superiorly, interiorly, anteriorly and posteriorly to the tip of the malleolus.

3 *cun* above the posterior border of tibia is Sanyinjiao (Sp. 6).

Zhaohai (K. 6) is directly below it, 0.4 *cun* below the inferior border the malleolus.

Zhongfeng (Liv. 4) is in front of the medial malleolus. Taixi (K. 3) is behind the medial malleolus.

The four points are all located with the tip of the malleolus as the landmark. (Fig. 43) (1), (2).

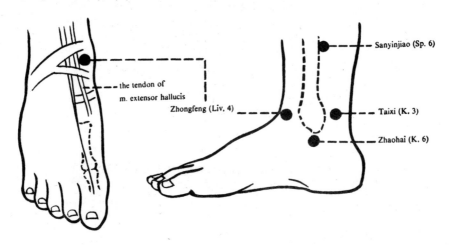

Fig. 43 Points Around Tip of the Malleolus

4. Leg: Points are located on the border of the tibia, on the bone surface and on the border of the tendon.

The border of the tibia: Sanyinjiao (Sp. 6) and Yinlingquan (Sp. 9) are on the posterior border of the tibia.

The bone surface: Ligou (Liv. 5) and Zhongdu (Liv. 6) are located on the middle of the medial surface of the tibia.

The border of the tendon: Fuliu (K. 7) and Zhubin (K. 9) are located anteriorly to the tendo calcaneus. (Fig. 44)

5. Knee joint: Points are located superiorly, inferiorly and posteriorly to the condyle.

The inferior part of the condyle: Yinlingquan (Sp. 9) is located on the inferior border of the medial condyle of the tibia, 1 *cun* posterior to Yinlingquan (Sp. 9) is Xiguan (Liv. 7). Yingu (K. 10) is posterior to Xiguan, between the two tendons, (of m. semitendinosus and semimembranosus).

The superior part of the condyle: Ququan (Liv. 8) is on the superior border of the medial epicondyle of the femur. (Fig. 45)

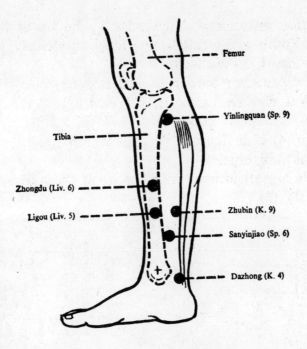

**Fig. 44 Points at Border and Surface of Tibia
and at Border of Achilles Tendon**

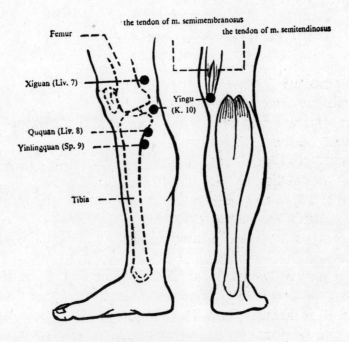

Fig. 45 Points near Condyle

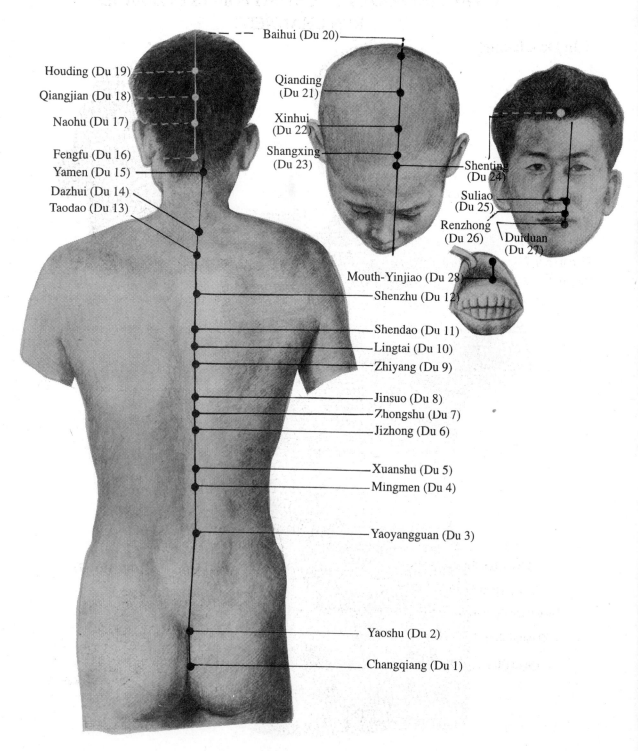

Houding (Du 19)
Qiangjian (Du 18)
Naohu (Du 17)
Fengfu (Du 16)
Yamen (Du 15)
Dazhui (Du 14)
Taodao (Du 13)

Baihui (Du 20)

Qianding (Du 21)

Xinhui (Du 22)

Shangxing (Du 23)

Shenting (Du 24)
Suliao (Du 25)
Renzhong (Du 26)
Duiduan (Du 27)

Mouth-Yinjiao (Du 28)
Shenzhu (Du 12)
Shendao (Du 11)
Lingtai (Du 10)
Zhiyang (Du 9)
Jinsuo (Du 8)
Zhongshu (Du 7)
Jizhong (Du 6)
Xuanshu (Du 5)
Mingmen (Du 4)
Yaoyangguan (Du 3)
Yaoshu (Du 2)
Changqiang (Du 1)

Fig. 46 The Du Channel

1.In Du Channel

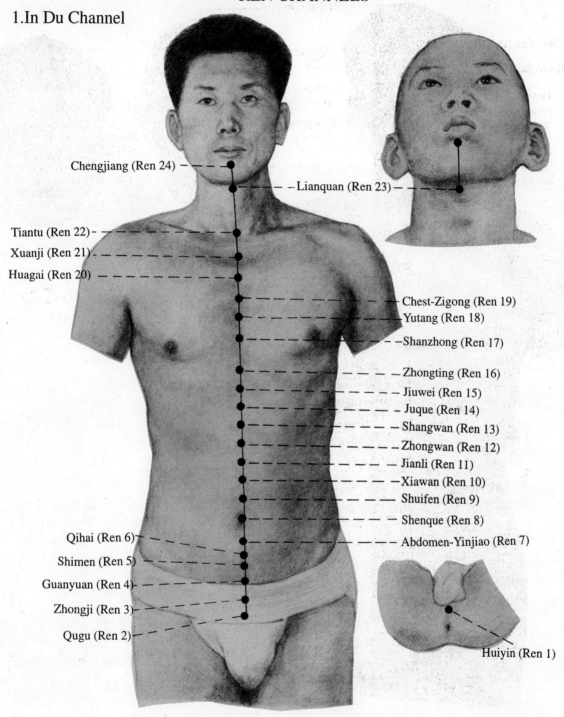

Chengjiang (Ren 24)

Lianquan (Ren 23)

Tiantu (Ren 22)

Xuanji (Ren 21)

Huagai (Ren 20)

Chest-Zigong (Ren 19)

Yutang (Ren 18)

Shanzhong (Ren 17)

Zhongting (Ren 16)

Jiuwei (Ren 15)

Juque (Ren 14)

Shangwan (Ren 13)

Zhongwan (Ren 12)

Jianli (Ren 11)

Xiawan (Ren 10)

Shuifen (Ren 9)

Shenque (Ren 8)

Qihai (Ren 6)

Shimen (Ren 5)

Guanyuan (Ren 4)

Zhongji (Ren 3)

Qugu (Ren 2)

Abdomen-Yinjiao (Ren 7)

Huiyin (Ren 1)

Fig. 47 The Ren Channel

The Du Channel starts at point Huiyin (Ren 1), goes upward along the midline of the lumbar, back, head and face, and ends at point Yinjiao (Du 28).

Changqiang (Du 1): Midway between the coccyx and the anus.

Yaoshu (Du 2): In the hiatus of the sacrum.

Except the 2nd, 4th, 8th, 12th thoracic and the 3rd lumbar vertebra there is a point below each of the spinous processes.

Yaoyangguan (Du 3): Below the spinous process of the 4th lumbar vertebra.

Mingmen (Du 4): Below the spinous process of the 2nd lumbar vertebra.

Xuanshu (Du 5): Below the spinous process of the 1st lumbar vertebra.

Jizhong (Du 6): Below the spinous process of the 11th thoracic vertebra.

Zhongshu (Du 7): Below the spinous process of the 10th thoracic vertebra.

Jinsuo (Du 8): Below the spinous process of the 9th thoracic vertebra.

Zhiyang (Du 9): Below the spinous process of the 7th thoracic vertebra.

Lingtai (Du 10): Below the spinous process of the 6th thoracic vertebra.

Shendao (Du 11): Below the spinous process of the 5th thoracic vertebra.

Shenzhu (Du 12): Below the spinous process of the 3rd thoracic vertabra.

Taodao (Du 13): Below the spinous process of the 1st thoracic vertebra.

Dazhui (Du 14): Between the spinous processes of the 7th cervical vertebra and the 1st thoracic vertebra.

Yamen (Du 15): At the midpoint of the nape, 0.5 *cun* above the posterior hairline.

Fengfu (Du 16): At the midpoint of the nape, 1 *cun* above the posterior hairline.

Naohu (Du 17): On the upper border of the occipital protuberance.

Qiangjian (Du 18): 1.5 *cun* above Naohu (Du 17).

Houding (Du 19): 1.5 *cun* above Qiangjian (Du 18).

Baihui (Du 20): Midpoint of the line connecting the two apexes of the ears.

Qianding (Du 21): 1.5 *cun* anterior to Baihui (Du 20).

Xinhui (Du 22): 1.5 *cun* anterior to Qianding (Du 21).

Shangxing (Du 23): 1 *cun* within the anterior hairline, on the midsagittal line of the head.

Shenting (Du 24): 0.5 *cun* within the anterior hairline, on the midsagittal line of the head.

Suliao (Du 25): On the tip of the nose.

Renzhong (Du 26): At the upper ⅓ of the philtrum.

Duiduan (Du 27): At the tip of the philtrum.

Yinjiao (Du 28): On the frenulum of the upper lip.

2. In Ren Channel

The Ren Channel starts at Huiyin (Ren 1), goes upward along the midline of the abdomen and the thorax and ends at Chengjiang (Ren 24), which is located below the lower lip.

Huiyin (Ren 1): In the centre of the perineum.

The distance between the umbilicus and the upper border of the pubis symphysis is 5 *cun*. The points located on the midline of the abdomen and are 1 *cun* apart, except for Qihai (Ren 6) which is 1.5 *cun* below the umbilicus.

Qugu (Ren 2): At the upper border of the symphysis pubis, on the midline of the abdomen.

Zhongji (Ren 3): 1 *cun* above Qugu (Ren 2).

Guanyuan (Ren 4): 1 *cun* above Zhongji (Ren 3).

Shimen (Ren 5): 1 *cun* above Guanyuan (Ren 4).

Qihai (Ren 6): 0.5 *cun* above Shimen (Ren 5).

Abdomen-Yinjiao (Ren 7): 0.5 *cun* above Qihai (Ren 6).

Shenque (Ren 8): In the centre of the umbilicus.

From the umbilicus to the lower border of the sternum is 8 *cun*. Between them, on the midline of abdomen, there are 8 points, each two being 1 *cun* apart. They are from the bottom to the top:

Shuifen (Ren 9): 1 *cun* above Shenque (Ren 8).

Xiawan (Ren 10): 1 *cun* above Shuifen (Ren 9).

Jianli (Ren 11): 1 *cun* above Xiawan (Ren 10).

Zhongwan (Ren 12): 1 *cun* above Jianli (Ren 11), 4 *cun* above the umbilicus.

Shangwan (Ren 13): 1 *cun* above Zhongwan (Ren 12).

Juque (Ren 14): 1 *cun* above Shangwan (Ren 13).

Jiuwei (Ren 15): 1 *cun* above Juque (Ren 14).

Zhongting (Ren 16): 1 *cun* above Jiuwei (Ren 15). Level with the lower border of the sternum body.

On the thorax, there are 6 points, all on the midsternal line, and they are 1 rib apart:

Shanzhong (Ren 17): It's located between the nipples, level with the 4th intercostal space.

Yutang (Ren 18): 1 rib above Shanzhong (Ren 17).

Chest-Zigong (Ren 19): 1 rib above Yutang (Ren 18).

Huagai (Ren 20): 1 rib above Chest-Zigong (Ren 19).

Xuanji (Ren 21): 1 rib above Huagai (Ren 20).

Tiantu (Ren 22): In the centre of the suprasternal fossa.

Lianquan (Ren 23): Between the Adam's apple and the mandible.

Chengjiang (Ren 24): In the depression under the lower lip.

VI. THE RULE OF LOCATING POINTS ON THE TRUNK

Rules for locating points on the lumbodorsal region: 1.5 *cun* and 3 *cun* lateral to the interspace between two vertebra. The points of the 1st line of the Urinary Bladder are located 1.5 *cun* lateral to the spinal column, and those of the 2nd line are 3 *cun* lateral to the spinal column.

Rules for locating points on the thoracic region: Midline of the thorax are points of the Ren Channel. 2 *cun* lateral to the Ren Channel are points of the Kidney Channel, 4 *cun* lateral to the Ren Channel are points of the Stomach Channel, and 5 *cun* lateral to the Ren Channel are points of the Lung and Spleen Channels. All these points are in the intercostal spaces.

Rules for locating points on the abdomen: Generally, points are 1 *cun* apart, and are 0.5, 2 or 4 *cun* lateral to the midline. 0.5 *cun* lateral to the midline are points of the Kidney Channel, 2 *cun* lateral to the midline are points of the Stomach Channel, and 4 *cun* lateral to the midline are points of the Spleen Channel.

Though there are a large number of points on the body, if you grasp the relative positions of the points of different channels in the same region and know how to make use of the anatomical landmarks on the body surface, you will be able to locate them accurately.

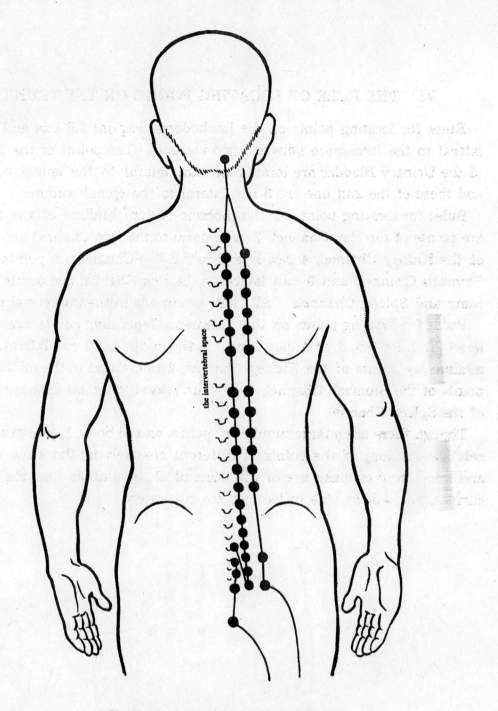

the intervetebral space

Fig. 48 1.5 or 3 Cun Lateral to Intervetebral Space

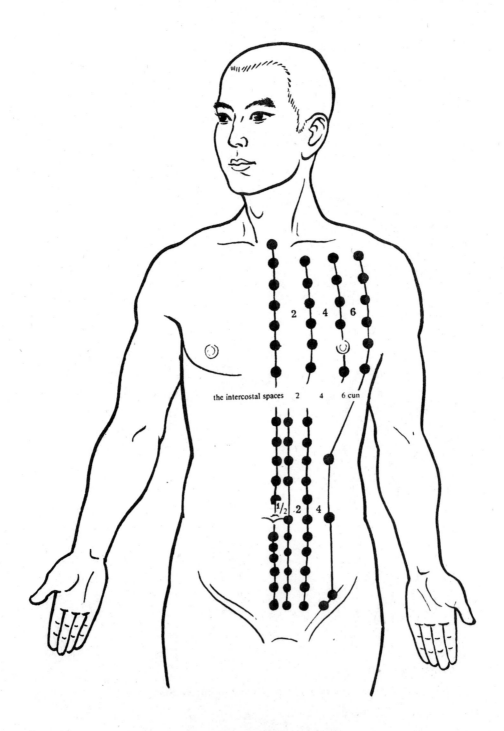

the intercostal spaces   2   4   6 cun

Fig. 49 1 Cun Superior and Inferior
1/2, 2, 4 Cun Lateral to Midline

图书在版编目(CIP)数据

针灸取穴法:英文/杨甲三编;孟宪坤,李学武译.—北京：
外文出版社,1998 重印
ISBN 7 - 119 - 00669 - X

Ⅰ.针… Ⅱ.①杨… ②孟… ③李… Ⅲ.针灸疗法－穴位－
基本知识－英文 Ⅳ.R244.2

中国版本图书馆 CIP 数据核字 (97) 第 09394 号

针灸取穴法

杨甲三　编

孟宪坤　李学武　译

何梅生　改稿

*

ⓒ外文出版社

外文出版社出版

（中国北京百万庄大街 24 号）

邮政编码 100037

北京外文印刷厂印刷

中国国际图书贸易总公司发行

（中国北京车公庄西路 35 号）

北京邮政信箱第 399 号　邮政编码 100044

1982 年(16 开)第 1 版

1998 年第 1 版第 3 次印刷

（英）

ISBN 7 - 119 - 00669 - X /R·15(外)

02000

14 - E - 1593P